Thyroid Truths

Hard-Earned Lessons from Hyperactive, Thyroidectomy, and Hypoactive Healing

Brin De Bellis

This book is designed to offer information and education. It is not intended to replace your relationship with your doctor, medical, or pharmaceutical professional, nor should it be used as a substitute for their guidance. The content does not constitute medical practice or advice. Neither the publisher, the author, any individuals mentioned or quoted, nor any of the medical, health, or wellness practitioners referenced in this book assume responsibility for any outcomes related to treatments, procedures, health modifications, or actions taken by readers based on the information provided.

Before starting any treatment or making modifications to your health regimen, the author and publisher strongly recommend consulting with your physician or medical professional. This includes discussing any prescription medications, vitamins, minerals, supplements, or other therapies to determine what is most appropriate and beneficial for your specific health needs and the correct dosages for you.

Every effort has been made to ensure this book is as thorough and accurate as possible. However, there may still be errors, both in content and typographical. Therefore, this book should be used as a guide and not considered the definitive source of information on thyroid, adrenal, or related health issues. Additionally, the information provided is current only as of the publication date.

Book design by Brin De Bellis
Cover design by Brin De Bellis

First Edition: October 2024

ISBN for Ebook : 978-1-7637433-0-4
ISBN for Paperback : 978-1-7637433-1-1

A Personal Journey of Struggle, Discovery, and Hope

When I was first diagnosed with a thyroid disorder, I had no idea how much my life was about to change. What began as a nagging collection of symptoms—fatigue, anxiety, and rapid weight changes—quickly spiralled into a confusing and often overwhelming journey through hyperthyroidism, surgery, and eventually life with an underactive thyroid. Along the way, I faced frustration with medical advice, uncertainty about my future, and a deep desire to regain control of my health.

But through the struggle came clarity. I realized that the key to living well with a thyroid condition isn't just about finding the right medication—it's about becoming informed, empowered, and proactive in your own care. This book is a reflection of my personal journey, the lessons I learned, and the practical tips that have made a real difference in my life.

Whether you're newly diagnosed or have been living with thyroid disease for years, my hope is that this book will provide you with guidance, encouragement, and the knowledge you need to thrive.

Introduction to My Thyroid Journey and what led me to write this book

Thyroid disease runs deep in my family. Both my mother and sisters have struggled with thyroid disorders, whether overactive or underactive. Yet, in my case, the condition seemed to be the most severe. Looking back now, I believe that the constant stress and challenges in my life played a major role in triggering and exacerbating my thyroid issues.

Before my diagnosis, I led a somewhat active lifestyle and never had to worry about my weight, even though I was quite thin. It wasn't until my early 20s, after becoming a mother, that the signs of thyroid dysfunction began to surface. Juggling the demands of a stressful marriage, raising a young daughter, studying for my master's degree, and adapting to a new country were overwhelming enough. But when I was diagnosed with an overactive thyroid— Graves' disease—it added another layer of complexity to my already stressful life.

For years, I tried to manage my condition with medication, but the constant pressure of life, work, and financial challenges made it difficult to find the time and space to truly focus on my health. After several years of struggling with hyperthyroidism, I eventually opted for a total thyroidectomy, hoping for a permanent solution. However, the years following the surgery brought new challenges as I transitioned to living with hypothyroidism.

Throughout my journey, I experienced the frustration of navigating the healthcare system, searching for the right treatment, and dealing with the emotional and physical toll of both thyroid conditions. From severe weight gain to mental health struggles, I found myself constantly searching for answers and solutions that traditional medicine didn't always provide.

I'm writing this book to share my experiences and the lessons I've learned along the way. I know firsthand how difficult it can be to find the right treatment, to advocate for yourself, and to manage the impact that thyroid disease can have on every aspect of your life. My hope is that by sharing my story, I can help others facing similar struggles feel less alone and more empowered to take control of their thyroid health.

This book is not just about my journey, but also a guide to help you navigate your own. Whether you're dealing with an overactive or underactive thyroid, or are somewhere in between, I hope the insights and practical tips I provide will help you along your path to healing and balance.

TABLE OF CONTENTS

Chapter 1: Understanding the Different Types of Thyroid Disorders

The thyroid, a small but powerful butterfly-shaped gland at the base of your neck, is the engine that powers many of the body's vital functions. Despite its size, when the thyroid malfunctions, it can affect nearly every system in the body, leaving a lasting impact on both physical and emotional well-being.

For many, thyroid disorders are mysterious and difficult to detect early on because their symptoms are often mistaken for other conditions. In this chapter, we'll dive into the most common thyroid disorders, breaking down how each one affects the body, the symptoms to look out for, and the treatment options available. Whether you're facing an overactive or underactive thyroid, knowing the nuances of each condition is the first step toward regaining control of your health.

1. Hypothyroidism (Underactive Thyroid)

Imagine your body's engine running slower than usual, making even the simplest tasks feel like they require more effort. That's what it's like living with hypothyroidism. This condition occurs when the thyroid fails to produce enough hormones, which slows down your body's metabolism.

- **Symptoms**: People with hypothyroidism often experience fatigue, unexplained weight gain, depression,

- dry skin, constipation, and increased sensitivity to cold. Daily life can feel exhausting, as your energy levels plummet and mental fog takes over.

- **Causes**: The most common cause is Hashimoto's thyroiditis, an autoimmune disorder where the body mistakenly attacks its own thyroid. Other causes include iodine deficiency, radiation treatment, and surgical removal of the thyroid.

- **Treatment**: Thankfully, hypothyroidism can often be managed effectively with thyroid hormone replacement therapy, which helps restore hormone levels to normal.

2. Hyperthyroidism (Overactive Thyroid)

Now imagine the opposite—a body that's constantly running in overdrive, where everything feels accelerated. This is hyperthyroidism, a condition where the thyroid produces too much hormone, speeding up your metabolism.

- **Symptoms**: Weight loss, rapid heartbeat, anxiety, tremors, sweating, and sensitivity to heat are common indicators. People with hyperthyroidism may feel jittery, like they can never fully relax, and struggle with insomnia or irritability.

- **Causes**: The most common culprit is Graves' disease, another autoimmune condition where the immune system overstimulates the thyroid. Other causes include thyroid nodules or inflammation of the thyroid (thyroiditis).

- **Treatment**: Treatments range from anti-thyroid medications and radioactive iodine therapy to thyroid surgery. These aim to slow down the thyroid's hormone production and restore balance.

3. Hashimoto's Thyroiditis

Hashimoto's thyroiditis is an autoimmune disorder in which the immune system attacks the thyroid gland, leading to chronic inflammation and eventually hypothyroidism. Over time, this leads to inflammation and gradual destruction of thyroid function. This is the most common cause of hypothyroidism and tends to develop slowly over time. Patients may not notice symptoms at first, but as the condition progresses, they may experience fatigue, weight gain, and depression.

- **Symptoms**: Early symptoms may be subtle, but as the condition progresses, fatigue, weight gain, depression, and a swollen thyroid (goiter) become more prominent.

- **Treatment**: Treatment typically involves thyroid hormone replacement to maintain normal levels of thyroid hormones in the body.

4. Graves' Disease

Graves' disease is an autoimmune condition that leads to hyperthyroidism. Graves' disease is the most common cause of hyperthyroidism and is a powerful example of how the immune system can wreak havoc on the thyroid. In Graves' disease, the immune system stimulates the thyroid to produce an excess of hormones. This condition is most common in women and can also cause eye problems, such as bulging eyes (Graves' ophthalmopathy) and, less commonly, skin issues (Graves' dermopathy).

- **Symptoms:** Anxiety, weight loss, increased heart rate, hand tremors, and bulging eyes (Graves' ophthalmopathy) are typical symptoms. The bulging eyes associated with Graves' disease can sometimes lead to vision problems and discomfort.

- **Treatment:** Anti-thyroid medications, radioactive iodine, or surgery to remove part or all of the thyroid are the most common treatments.

5. Goiter

Goiter is an abnormal enlargement of the thyroid gland. It is not a disease itself but a symptom of various thyroid conditions, including hypothyroidism, hyperthyroidism, or iodine deficiency. In many cases, a goiter may not cause symptoms but can lead to difficulty swallowing, coughing, or discomfort in the neck.

- **Symptoms:** A noticeable swelling in the neck, difficulty swallowing, coughing, and a tight feeling in the throat may develop as the goiter grows.
- **Treatment:** Depending on the cause, treatment may involve iodine supplements, thyroid hormone replacement, or surgery to remove the enlarged gland.

6. Thyroid Nodules

Thyroid nodules are lumps or growths within the thyroid gland. Most nodules are benign (non-cancerous), but some can be cancerous. They may cause symptoms such as difficulty swallowing or breathing, but many are discovered incidentally during a physical exam or imaging tests for unrelated issues. Nodules can sometimes produce excess thyroid hormone, leading to hyperthyroidism.

- **Symptoms**: Often asymptomatic, but large nodules may cause difficulty swallowing or breathing. Some nodules may cause hyperthyroid symptoms.
- **Treatment**: Monitoring, biopsy, or surgery may be required based on the size and nature of the nodule. Radioactive iodine may be used in cases where the nodules are overproducing hormones.

7. Thyroid Cancer

Thyroid cancer occurs when malignant cells form in the tissues of the thyroid gland. It is relatively rare but is more common in women. Most thyroid cancers are treatable and have a good prognosis. There are several types of thyroid cancer, including papillary, follicular, medullary, and anaplastic. Symptoms may include a lump in the neck, hoarseness, and difficulty swallowing.

- **Symptoms**: A lump in the neck, changes in voice, difficulty swallowing, and swollen lymph nodes may be signs of thyroid cancer. While these symptoms can seem similar to benign thyroid disorders, they warrant immediate medical attention.

- **Treatment**: Surgery is the most common treatment, often followed by radioactive iodine therapy, radiation, or chemotherapy depending on the type and stage of the cancer.

A Complex System with Unique Challenges

The thyroid gland, though small, governs an intricate system that impacts nearly every part of the body. From regulating metabolism to controlling how fast or slow your organs function, the thyroid is a powerhouse that often goes unnoticed—until something goes wrong. Understanding the various types of thyroid disorders is crucial because each one affects the body in very distinct ways. The treatment plans, the symptoms, and the path to healing can vary greatly, not only from condition to condition but also from person to person. This individuality is what makes thyroid disorders so complex—and so challenging.

As you dive deeper into this book, you'll come to see that managing a thyroid disorder is not just about taking medication or following a standard protocol. It's about understanding your unique body, your unique challenges, and finding a treatment plan that fits you as an individual. In the chapters ahead, I will walk you through my personal experience with both **hyperthyroidism** and **hypothyroidism**, shedding light on what it feels like to live at both extremes. Through my journey, I've learned valuable lessons— lessons that I hope will not only resonate with you but also provide practical insights for managing your own thyroid health.

If you suspect that something might be off with your thyroid, don't hesitate to seek help. The earlier you address it, the better your chances of managing the condition effectively. The thyroid may be small, but the effect it has on your overall health is profound. Early detection can make a world of difference, as the longer a thyroid disorder goes undiagnosed, the more it can disrupt your daily life, affecting not just your physical body but also your mental and emotional well-being.

When you look at the broad spectrum of thyroid disorders, it becomes clear that most of them can be categorized into two primary types: **overactive (hyperthyroidism)** and **underactive (hypothyroidism)**. These two conditions might seem like opposites—and in many ways, they are—but they both come with their own unique set of challenges. They impact not only the physical body but also the mind and spirit, in ways that are difficult to fully comprehend unless you've experienced them firsthand.

For many, the road to a thyroid diagnosis can be long and frustrating. Symptoms can be subtle at first, easy to dismiss or misattribute to stress or aging. However, as the condition worsens, the effects become more noticeable and harder to ignore. Whether you're feeling like your body is always in overdrive or as if you're constantly running on empty, the thyroid plays a central role in how you feel day-to-day.

My personal journey with thyroid disease took me through both extremes. I started with hyperthyroidism, a condition where my body felt as though it was perpetually stuck in high gear. My heart raced, I couldn't quiet my mind, and my energy levels swung wildly from bursts of nervous energy to overwhelming fatigue. It felt like I was constantly being pulled in different directions, struggling to balance the demands of everyday life while my body ran on overdrive. Every small task felt like an urgent deadline, and stress became a constant companion.

Living with hyperthyroidism was like trying to control a speeding car that had no brakes. My body was running too fast for its own good, and the constant influx of thyroid hormones left me feeling drained and jittery. My mind rarely felt at ease, my emotions were volatile, and the physical symptoms—like weight loss, heart palpitations, and hot flashes—were difficult to manage. The confusion and stress compounded, as I tried to figure out how to regain control of my life and my health.

After years of managing hyperthyroidism, I experienced a shift that was equally challenging, but in the opposite direction: hypothyroidism. Suddenly, my body wasn't racing anymore—it was slowing down. Things that once seemed easy now required enormous effort. Simple tasks became exhausting, and the weight that I had once struggled to keep off began to pile on. The mental fog that accompanies hypothyroidism was perhaps one of the hardest symptoms to cope with. My mind, once sharp and alert, felt dulled. I struggled to focus, to concentrate, and to maintain the energy needed for everyday life.

In contrast to hyperthyroidism, where I felt constantly "wired," hypothyroidism made me feel like I was wading through mud. The fatigue was overwhelming, my muscles ached, and my metabolism slowed to a crawl. The emotional impact of this shift was profound. I went from feeling anxious and overstimulated to feeling sluggish, depressed, and often hopeless. It was as though my body had betrayed me, swinging from one extreme to another, never quite finding balance.

Having lived through both of these conditions, I've gained a deep understanding of what it means to have your body constantly shifting between these extremes. Each condition comes with its own unique challenges, and the way you treat one is vastly different from the way you treat the other. Hyperthyroidism requires a delicate balancing act of slowing down the thyroid, while hypothyroidism involves boosting it. Through a lot of trial and error, frustration, and perseverance, I've learned what works—and what doesn't—when it comes to managing both conditions.

This book is my way of sharing those hard-earned insights. Whether you're experiencing the rapid-fire symptoms of an overactive thyroid or the sluggish, exhausting effects of an underactive one, I understand the frustration, the confusion, and the uncertainty you may be facing. I know what it feels like to be on both sides of the spectrum, and I know that finding balance can seem like an impossible task.

But healing is possible. The process for each condition is different, and there is no one-size-fits-all approach. My hope is that by sharing my journey, you'll find something that resonates with you—whether it's a treatment option you haven't yet considered, a lifestyle change that can make a difference, or simply the reassurance that you are not alone in this struggle. I've walked both paths, and through my own experience, I've learned the best ways to support the body, mind, and spirit when dealing with thyroid disease.

Navigating thyroid health can feel overwhelming, but it doesn't have to be a battle you face alone. My journey taught me that there is strength in knowledge, power in self-advocacy, and healing in perseverance. As you move through this book, I hope you'll gain not only a deeper understanding of thyroid disorders but also the confidence and tools to take control of your health. My wish for you is that, by the end of this journey, you'll have found a path toward balance, peace, and well-being in your own thyroid health.

Chapter 2: The Battle Begins – Living with Hyperthyroidism

Life has a way of presenting challenges that test not only your strength but also your resolve. Becoming a mother at the age of 26 was one of the most rewarding moments of my life, but it also marked the beginning of a turbulent chapter. While my beautiful daughter filled me with joy, the stress and strain from an unstable marriage, the financial burdens, and the challenge of balancing education, work, and motherhood took a heavy toll. What I didn't realize at the time was that my body was struggling under the weight of hyperthyroidism—an invisible battle that would only reveal itself after a series of health scares.

New Chapter: Motherhood and Health Struggles

Looking back, it's clear that the stress of my marriage was a major factor in my deteriorating health. My husband at the time was dealing with mental illness, combined with his issues of gambling and infidelity, had created an unstable home environment. This emotional turmoil, coupled with the demands of caring for a newborn, was overwhelming. On top of it all, I was pursuing a master's degree in accounting, trying to secure a stable future for my daughter and myself. Juggling these responsibilities felt like I was always on the edge, and while I knew I was tired and stressed, I never imagined that something more serious was happening within my body.

Migrating to Australia at the age of 24 meant I had to rebuild my life from the ground up. With no established network and a marriage that wasn't providing the support I needed, I was running on fumes, both emotionally and physically. It was during this chaos that my mother noticed something unusual - a swelling on my neck, which we later learned was a goiter. This moment was a turning point. Although I had been experiencing fatigue, irritability, and weight fluctuations, I had attributed it all to the stress I was under. However, my mother's observation led me to visit a doctor, and that's when the true nature of my health condition was revealed.

Hyperthyroidism: What It Means and How It Affects the Body

After undergoing a series of tests, including blood work and a physical examination of my neck, the doctor confirmed that I had **hyperthyroidism**, more specifically **Graves' disease**. This autoimmune disorder was causing my thyroid gland to produce excessive hormones, sending my metabolism into overdrive. Graves' disease is the most common cause of hyperthyroidism, affecting millions of people worldwide, particularly women.

When you have hyperthyroidism, your body's engine is constantly revving, even when you're at rest. Imagine a car stuck in the highest gear, speeding along without the ability to slow down. That's what hyperthyroidism does to your body—it pushes every function into overdrive, which is why common symptoms include **unexplained weight loss, rapid heartbeat, anxiety, and excessive sweating**. For someone like me, already dealing with high levels of stress, this diagnosis felt like another burden to carry, but one I couldn't ignore.

In a normal, healthy body, the thyroid gland produces hormones—**thyroxine (T4)** and **triiodothyronine (T3)**—that help regulate metabolism, heart rate, and energy levels. These hormones ensure that your body functions optimally, keeping everything from your digestion to your heartbeat in check. When the thyroid produces too much T4 and T3, as it does in hyperthyroidism, it throws your entire system into chaos.

Hyperthyroidism affects roughly **1 in 100 people**, and while many cases are manageable, the symptoms can vary widely. For me, it meant that my weight, which had always been stable, dropped drastically. I had always been small, with an optimal weight of around **56 kg (123 pounds)**, but I quickly fell below 50 kg (**110 pounds**), becoming increasingly frail. This weight loss, while alarming to those around me, wasn't something I focused on initially. In fact, part of me was grateful for not having to worry about my weight at a time when everything else in my life was so overwhelming.

The Financial and Emotional Toll of Treatment

Following my diagnosis, I began antithyroid medication, specifically **methimazole**, which is commonly prescribed to help slow down the thyroid's overproduction of hormones. This medication was supposed to bring balance to my hormone levels, but it came with its own set of challenges. The most immediate challenge was the financial burden. Every two weeks, I had to undergo blood tests to monitor my hormone levels and adjust my medication dosage accordingly. Each doctor's visit, each test, and every consultation with a specialist cost money—money that I didn't always have.

At the time, I was already struggling to manage my finances while studying and caring for a baby. The constant medical expenses were overwhelming, and I often had to choose between my health and other essentials. This is a reality many people with chronic conditions face—the dilemma of prioritizing health in the midst of financial hardship. For three years, from **2014 to 2017**, I was in and out of the doctor's office, trying to find the right balance of treatment. Some days, the medication worked well, and my symptoms were manageable. On other days, the side effects were almost as debilitating as the illness itself.

On top of the financial strain, there was the emotional toll. Living with a chronic illness like hyperthyroidism is mentally exhausting. The unpredictability of my symptoms, the constant doctor visits, and the pressure to maintain some sense of normalcy weighed heavily on me. I was raising a young child, studying for a degree, and navigating a failing marriage, all while my body was fighting an invisible battle. The emotional fatigue often felt harder to manage than the physical symptoms.

The Compounding Effects of Stress

Stress, as I learned the hard way, has a direct impact on thyroid health, especially in cases of hyperthyroidism. Research has shown that stress can exacerbate symptoms of Graves' disease and even trigger flare-ups. When you're already dealing with an overactive thyroid, the additional cortisol—your body's stress hormone—only fuels the fire. I was living in a state of perpetual stress, which made managing my hyperthyroidism even more difficult.

In my case, stress manifested in heart palpitations, anxiety, and hot flushes. There were moments when my heart would race uncontrollably, leaving me feeling like I had run a marathon, even when I was sitting still. The hot flushes were perhaps the most unsettling. At work, under the pressure of tight deadlines, I would feel my body temperature spike suddenly, my face flushed, and sweat would begin to pour. These episodes made it difficult to focus, and worse, they made me feel out of control. The **external stress** from my job and personal life was compounding the **internal stress** of my illness, creating a vicious cycle.

For someone working in a high-pressure environment like auditor at the time, where precision and focus are key, this was a disaster. The constant need to meet deadlines, the long hours, and the pressure to perform at a high level only worsened my condition. I often found myself snapping at colleagues or becoming frustrated over small things—behaviors that were completely out of character for me. It was as if my body and mind were no longer my own.

The Emotional Rollercoaster of Hyperthyroidism

Hyperthyroidism doesn't just take a toll on the body—it wreaks havoc on the mind. The hormonal imbalance caused by an overactive thyroid can lead to **mood swings, irritability, and even depression**. For me, these emotional ups and downs were some of the hardest parts of living with the condition. One moment, I'd feel incredibly anxious and restless, unable to sit still or focus. The next, I'd feel overwhelmed with sadness or frustration, often losing my temper over things that normally wouldn't bother me.

These mood swings affected my ability to be present for my daughter, which was heartbreaking. I wanted to be the calm, loving mother she deserved, but instead, I often felt short-tempered and irritable. The guilt that came with these feelings was immense. I knew that much of my behavior was out of my control, driven by the hormonal chaos happening inside me, but that didn't make it any easier to bear.

I also found that hyperthyroidism affected my memory and concentration. This is a lesser-known symptom, but for many people with overactive thyroids, "**brain fog**" is a real and frustrating issue. I would forget important tasks, struggle to concentrate on my studies, and even lose track of conversations. It felt as though my mind was constantly running too fast to keep up with itself, leaving me in a state of perpetual mental exhaustion.

The Long Road to Acceptance

For three long years, I tried to manage my condition with medication, lifestyle changes, and regular monitoring. The results were mixed. While the antithyroid medication helped to control some of my symptoms, it wasn't a permanent solution. The constant blood tests, medication adjustments, and unpredictable flare-ups left me feeling like I was stuck in a never-ending cycle.

By **2017**, I had reached a breaking point. I knew I needed a more permanent solution. My body, already worn down by years of hyperthyroidism, stress, and emotional exhaustion, couldn't take much more. After consulting with my doctors, I made the difficult decision to undergo a **total thyroidectomy**—the complete removal of my thyroid gland. It wasn't an easy choice, but at that point, I was desperate for relief.

Looking Back: Lessons Learned from Hyperthyroidism

As I reflect on my journey with hyperthyroidism, I realize how much I've learned—not just about the condition itself, but about the importance of self-care, stress management, and advocating for one's health. Hyperthyroidism may be a medical condition, but its impact goes far beyond physical symptoms. It affects every aspect of life— mental, emotional, and even social.

If I could go back, I would have taken more time to explore **natural methods** for managing my condition, such as stress reduction techniques, dietary changes, and holistic therapies. There is growing evidence that these approaches can complement traditional medical treatments, helping to reduce symptoms and improve overall well-being. But at the time, I was simply in survival mode, doing my best to keep everything together.

Ultimately, hyperthyroidism taught me the importance of listening to my body and seeking help when I need it. It's a condition that requires constant vigilance, but it's also one that can be managed with the right combination of medical treatment, self-care, and support.

Chapter 3: The Decision to Undergo Thyroidectomy

By 2018, I had been living with the unpredictable nature of hyperthyroidism for several years. The constant back-and-forth of taking antithyroid medication, getting my hormone levels tested, adjusting my treatment, and then starting the whole cycle over again was draining, both physically and emotionally. I had tried so hard to manage my condition, but it felt like a losing battle. The moments when my symptoms eased were fleeting, and the inevitable flare-ups were exhausting. I knew I couldn't continue living like that—I needed a permanent solution, something that would bring an end to the turmoil.

I was at a crossroads. The idea of continuing with temporary treatments, knowing they weren't providing lasting relief, filled me with anxiety. I wanted to take back control of my health, to find a way out of the constant uncertainty that came with hyperthyroidism. My body had become a battleground, and I felt as though I was losing the fight. The palpitations, the hot flashes, the weight fluctuations, and the erratic mood swings had left me feeling vulnerable and worn down. The decision to seek a more permanent solution was driven by a deep need to regain stability in my life.

The decision to explore more permanent solutions was not made lightly. I spent countless hours researching my options, talking to my doctors, and contemplating the long-term effects of each treatment. The choice I faced was between two major treatments—**radioactive iodine therapy (RAI)** or **total thyroidectomy**. Each option carried its own risks and benefits, and neither was an easy choice.

Weighing the Options: Radioactive Iodine vs. Thyroidectomy

Both treatments promised the same result—eliminating the overactive thyroid—but they approached it in very different ways. Radioactive iodine therapy, or RAI, involves swallowing a small amount of radioactive iodine, which is absorbed by the thyroid gland and destroys the overactive cells. This option seemed appealing because it was non-invasive. There was no need for surgery, no recovery time, and it was generally considered effective. However, as I delved deeper into my research, the idea of using radiation to treat my thyroid made me uncomfortable. While it targeted the thyroid, there was a risk that the radiation could affect other tissues in the body, and I wasn't willing to take that chance. I worried about the long-term effects, about what might happen if the radiation damaged other parts of my body. RAI felt too unpredictable for my peace of mind.

The other option was total thyroidectomy, the surgical removal of the entire thyroid gland. This was a more aggressive approach, involving a physical operation and the permanent loss of my thyroid. The upside was that it offered a definitive solution—once the thyroid was removed, there would be no more fluctuations in hormone levels. The downside, however, was that I would be left completely dependent on thyroid hormone replacement for the rest of my life. Thyroidectomy is a major surgery, and like any surgery, it came with risks—potential damage to the vocal cords, nerves, or parathyroid glands.

It wasn't an easy decision. I spent weeks pouring over research, reading personal stories of people who had undergone both treatments, and weighing the pros and cons. I talked to my endocrinologist, who explained the benefits and risks of each option. He was a patient and knowledgeable doctor, but even he couldn't give me the definitive answer I was searching for. Ultimately, the choice was mine.

A Personal Fear: Protecting My Eyes

One of the main reasons I ultimately leaned toward surgery was a deeply personal fear: the possibility of Graves' ophthalmopathy. With Graves' disease, there's a risk that the eyes can start to protrude—a condition known as exophthalmos. It's caused by the swelling of muscles and tissues behind the eyes, which pushes them forward, creating a bulging effect. For me, this was terrifying. I had begun to notice subtle changes in my eyes—they were slightly more prominent, and they felt irritated and dry. While the protrusion hadn't become severe, I could see the early signs, and it shook me to my core.

The idea of living with bulging eyes was devastating to me. I knew that once Graves' ophthalmopathy took hold, it could be difficult—if not impossible—to reverse, even with treatment. The thought of my appearance changing so drastically, of my eyes protruding in a way that would forever alter how I looked, filled me with dread. I didn't want to live with that fear, constantly worrying that my condition would progress to the point of no return. For many people, the cosmetic effects of eye bulging may seem trivial in the grand scheme of things, but for me, it was deeply emotional. My eyes are such a central part of who I am—how I connect with the world, how I express myself. I couldn't imagine losing that.

This fear, more than anything else, tipped the scales in favor of surgery. I knew that removing my thyroid would eliminate the source of the problem and, hopefully, prevent my eyes from worsening. While the surgery itself came with its own set of risks, it felt like the more certain option—one that would give me back some semblance of control over my body and my future.

The Decision: Opting for Surgery

After much soul-searching, I decided to move forward with the total thyroidectomy. I was looking for a long-term solution, something that would allow me to put the uncertainty behind me and move forward with my life. Radioactive iodine felt too unpredictable, and I couldn't shake the feeling that radiation could cause damage elsewhere in my body. Surgery seemed like the more definitive option, even though it was permanent and came with its own set of challenges.

It wasn't just a medical decision—it was an emotional one. I would lose a part of my body that, while causing problems, was still an essential organ. The thyroid is a small but mighty gland, regulating so many vital functions in the body. I had come to understand just how crucial it was through my experience with hyperthyroidism, and the thought of losing it forever was daunting. There were moments when I doubted my decision, moments when I wished I could find another way to heal my thyroid naturally.

If I could go back and do it all over again, I would have explored natural treatments more thoroughly. I would have taken the time to detox my body, cleanse my system, and find ways to support my thyroid's natural function. I would have sought out holistic approaches, such as reducing stress through yoga and meditation, making dietary changes, and addressing the root causes of my thyroid imbalance. But in the whirlwind of life—juggling a child, a job, and managing a chronic illness—I didn't have the time, the knowledge, or the resources to explore those options fully. Surgery felt like the only way out.

I knew the decision would change my life, but I don't think I fully realized just how much it would. The surgery wasn't just a medical procedure—it was a turning point in my life, one that would set me on a new path, one where I would have to learn to live without my thyroid and rely on synthetic hormones for the rest of my life.

Preparing for Surgery: The Emotional Journey

In the weeks leading up to the surgery, I found myself going through a range of emotions—fear, hope, uncertainty, and even grief. I knew that the surgery was supposed to bring relief, but the reality of losing a part of my body was difficult to process. My thyroid, despite all the trouble it had caused, was still a part of me, and the thought of having it removed felt like I was losing a part of my identity.

I began to prepare myself mentally and physically for the surgery. I took pictures of my neck, knowing that after the operation, I would be left with a scar. It felt like a goodbye, in a way—saying farewell to the body I had known for so many years. I imagined what it would be like to look in the mirror after the surgery and see a permanent reminder of what I had been through. The scar would be small, but it would be there forever, a visible sign of the journey I had been on.

I spent a lot of time reflecting on what life would be like post-surgery. I imagined what it would feel like to wake up without the constant anxiety of hyperthyroidism, without the fear of my eyes protruding further. I tried to focus on the positives. I told myself that this surgery would bring me peace, that it would free me from the constant struggle of managing my hyperthyroidism. But there was still a sense of loss, a sense of uncertainty about what life would be like after the surgery. Would I feel better? Would I regret my decision? Would I be able to live without my thyroid?

The Day of the Surgery: Trusting the Process

On the day of the surgery, I was both anxious and ready. I had done my research, talked to my doctors, and made peace with my decision. My endocrinologist referred me to a skilled surgeon, one with years of experience performing thyroidectomies. While I was nervous about the procedure, I trusted that I was in good hands. The surgery would take place in a public Medicare hospital, and despite the fact that I wasn't paying for a private service, I felt confident that I would receive excellent care.

The surgery itself went smoothly. When I woke up in the recovery room, there was a sense of relief. It was done—the thyroid that had caused so much turmoil in my life was gone. My neck was bandaged, and I was sore, but I felt a sense of calm that I hadn't experienced in years. The worst was behind me. My eyes would be safe, and I wouldn't have to live in fear of their protruding further. That, alone, was a weight off my shoulders.

I spent the next few days recovering in the hospital, adjusting to life without my thyroid. My doctors started me on **levothyroxine**, a synthetic form of thyroid hormone that would replace the hormones my body could no longer produce. At first, I was put on a relatively low dose—**50 mcg**—which was gradually increased to **100 mcg** as my body adjusted to the change. It was strange to think that for the rest of my life, I would be dependent on this little pill to keep my body functioning properly. There was a new normal to adjust to, and while I was grateful for the success of the surgery, I also realized that this was only the beginning of a new chapter.

Life After Thyroidectomy: A New Normal

The weeks following the surgery were a blur of recovery and adjustment. Physically, I healed quickly. The scar on my neck, though visible, was smaller than I had feared, and over time, it would fade into something barely noticeable. But emotionally, the adjustment was more difficult. While I was relieved to be free from the constant fluctuations of hyperthyroidism, I now had to learn to live with hypothyroidism, a condition I had never fully prepared for.

Living without a thyroid meant that my body no longer had the ability to regulate its own hormone levels. I was entirely dependent on levothyroxine to keep my metabolism, energy, and overall health in balance. The medication worked well at first, and for a while, I felt like I was getting my life back. But as the months went by, I started to notice changes in my body that I hadn't anticipated—weight gain, fatigue, and mood swings. It became clear that finding the right dose of thyroid hormone replacement would be an ongoing process, one that required patience and careful monitoring.

Looking Back: Reflections on Thyroidectomy

If I were given another chance, would I have made a different decision? It's a question I ask myself often. Knowing what I know now, I would have taken more time to explore alternative treatments, to detox my body, reduce stress, and see if there was a way to heal my thyroid naturally. But at the time, surgery seemed like the best option—the only option, really.

I've come to accept that the decision I made was the right one for me at that moment in time. The thyroidectomy gave me freedom from the constant battle of hyperthyroidism, even if it came with its own set of challenges. While I may never know what life would have been like if I had kept my thyroid, I've learned to embrace the journey I'm on, scars and all.

The journey to thyroidectomy wasn't just a medical one—it was emotional, spiritual, and deeply personal. Losing my thyroid changed my life in ways I couldn't have anticipated, but it also freed me from the unpredictability of hyperthyroidism and the fear of what might happen to my eyes. In many ways, the surgery gave me a second chance at health, even if it came with its own set of challenges.

As I continue to navigate life without a thyroid, I've come to understand that healing is not always a straight line. It's a journey that requires patience, perseverance, and a willingness to adapt. While my decision to undergo a thyroidectomy changed my life forever, it also taught me the importance of listening to my body, advocating for my health, and trusting that I have the strength to face whatever challenges come my way.

Living without a thyroid means constant vigilance—regular blood tests, medication adjustments, and learning to listen to my body in new ways. It's not easy, but it's my new reality, and I've learned to adapt. The scar on my neck has faded over time, but it remains a reminder of the journey I've been through. Every time I look in the mirror, I'm reminded of the strength it took to make such a life-altering decision and the resilience that has carried me through.

Chapter 4: Life After Thyroidectomy – The Shift to Hypothyroidism

The thyroidectomy was meant to bring relief, a much-needed end to the unpredictability of hyperthyroidism. For years, I had battled the erratic symptoms of an overactive thyroid—heart palpitations, anxiety, weight loss, and emotional instability. The surgery felt like a final, decisive step toward regaining control over my health, and in some ways, it was. I no longer had to worry about my thyroid fluctuating wildly between extremes. The overactivity was gone. But what I didn't fully grasp at the time was that by removing my thyroid, I was entering a new and equally challenging phase of my journey—hypothyroidism.

Living without a thyroid meant I had permanently shifted from one extreme to the other, and the transition was anything but smooth. The thyroid, as small as it is, plays an enormous role in regulating metabolism, energy, and overall bodily functions. Without it, my body could no longer produce the hormones it needed to function properly, and I was now entirely reliant on **levothyroxine**, a synthetic form of thyroid hormone, to keep me going. What I didn't expect, though, was how difficult it would be to find the right balance. The shift from hyperthyroidism to hypothyroidism was not just a medical adjustment—it was a profound physical and emotional transformation.

The Immediate Aftermath: Adjusting to Hypothyroidism

In the weeks following the surgery, I was prescribed **50 mcg** of levothyroxine, which was later increased to **100 mcg** as my doctors worked to stabilize my hormone levels. Initially, I didn't feel the effects of the shift as strongly. My body was still recovering from the surgery, and I was relieved to be free from the hyperactivity that had plagued me for so long. The days of racing thoughts, sleepless nights, and constant anxiety were behind me, and for the first time in years, I felt a sense of calm.

But as the months passed, I began to realize that life without a thyroid presented its own set of challenges. While hyperthyroidism had left me feeling like my body was always in overdrive, hypothyroidism was the complete opposite. I went from feeling wired and anxious to feeling like I was moving through life in slow motion. Simple tasks that had once felt effortless now required enormous effort. My energy levels plummeted, and I found myself exhausted after even the smallest activities.

The weight I had struggled to keep off during hyperthyroidism began to creep back on. At first, it was just a few pounds, but as the months wore on, I gained more and more weight. For someone who had always been small-built, the steady increase in my weight was disheartening. I had gained over **12 kg (26 pounds)** within three years after the surgery, and my body no longer felt like my own. My clothes no longer fit, and I felt sluggish, heavy, and uncomfortable in my skin.

What I didn't realize at the time was that finding the right dose of levothyroxine was an ongoing process. The body's needs change over time, and adjusting to synthetic thyroid hormones is not a one-time fix. It requires constant monitoring, regular blood tests, and a delicate balance of medication. Too little hormone, and I would feel the effects of hypothyroidism—fatigue, weight gain, depression. Too much, and I risked tipping back into hyperthyroidism. The goal was to find that sweet spot, but it wasn't easy, and it required a level of patience I wasn't prepared for.

The Physical Consequences: A New Set of Challenges

Physically, the shift to hypothyroidism presented new challenges that were just as difficult—if not more so—than those I had faced with hyperthyroidism. One of the most frustrating symptoms was the overwhelming **fatigue**. No matter how much I rested, I never seemed to feel truly refreshed. Mornings were the hardest. Waking up felt like dragging myself through thick fog, and it often took hours before I could muster the energy to start my day. Even simple tasks, like getting dressed or making breakfast, felt like monumental efforts.

The weight gain was another difficult aspect to accept. During hyperthyroidism, I had been able to eat whatever I wanted without worrying about gaining weight. But now, my metabolism had slowed to a crawl. Despite eating healthy and maintaining an active lifestyle, the pounds kept piling on. It felt as though my body was working against me, no matter what I did. I would look in the mirror and barely recognize the person staring back. My small frame had become heavier, and with each passing month, I felt more out of control.

But the physical consequences weren't limited to fatigue and weight gain. I also experienced **joint and muscle pain**, something I hadn't anticipated. My body ached in ways it never had before. My feet would swell after standing for too long, and I could barely stand in the shower for more than a few minutes without feeling intense discomfort. This new level of pain was unfamiliar and unsettling, and I struggled to understand why my body was reacting this way.

The Emotional Consequences: Navigating Mental Health

If the physical symptoms of hypothyroidism were difficult, the emotional consequences were even harder to manage. One of the most challenging aspects of living with an underactive thyroid is the profound impact it has on mental health. With hyperthyroidism, I had experienced anxiety, restlessness, and irritability. But with hypothyroidism, it was **depression** and **mental fog** that took center stage.

There were days when I felt like I was walking around in a haze, unable to focus or concentrate. My once-sharp mind felt dulled, and tasks that required mental clarity—like studying or working—became nearly impossible. It was as if my brain had slowed down along with my body, and I couldn't shake the sense of lethargy that followed me everywhere. The mental fog made it difficult to stay organized, remember important details, and complete even the simplest tasks. I found myself forgetting things, losing track of time, and feeling overwhelmed by tasks that I used to handle with ease.

The **emotional toll** was just as heavy. Depression crept in slowly, but once it took hold, it was hard to shake. I felt weighed down not just physically, but emotionally as well. I struggled to find joy in the things I once loved, and the emotional swings left me feeling disconnected from myself and others. It was a stark contrast to the hyperactivity of Graves' disease. Instead of feeling like I was running on overdrive, I now felt like I was running on empty. And the hardest part was that I couldn't see a way out.

Hypothyroidism also affected my **self-esteem**. The weight gain, the sluggishness, and the constant feeling of being tired left me feeling unattractive and insecure. I didn't feel like myself anymore, and that sense of disconnect from my body only deepened my emotional struggles. It was hard to explain to others what I was going through. On the outside, it looked like I was just gaining weight or feeling tired, but on the inside, it felt like my entire world had been turned upside down.

Learning to Manage Hypothyroidism: Finding Balance

As the months passed, I began to realize that living with hypothyroidism required a whole new approach to managing my health. It wasn't enough to rely solely on medication. I had to become more attuned to my body's needs and make adjustments in all areas of my life. I started by focusing on my diet. I researched foods that could support thyroid health and tried to avoid processed foods that could slow down my already sluggish metabolism. I introduced more nutrient-dense foods, like leafy greens, lean proteins, and foods rich in selenium and zinc, which are known to support thyroid function.

Exercise also became an important part of my routine, though it wasn't easy at first. The fatigue and joint pain made it difficult to stay active, but I knew that staying sedentary would only make things worse. I started slowly, incorporating gentle forms of exercise like walking and yoga, and gradually built up my stamina. Movement helped not only with my physical symptoms but also with my mental health. On the days when I felt depressed or overwhelmed, even a short walk could lift my mood and clear my mind.

Perhaps the biggest lesson I learned during this time was the importance of patience. Hypothyroidism is not something that can be fixed overnight. It's a lifelong condition that requires ongoing management and adjustment. Finding the right dose of thyroid hormone replacement took time, and even then, it wasn't always perfect. I had to learn to listen to my body, to recognize when something was off, and to communicate with my doctors to make the necessary changes.

Reflections: Accepting a New Reality

Living with hypothyroidism is not what I had imagined when I underwent the thyroidectomy. I had hoped for a clean break from the chaos of hyperthyroidism, but what I found was a new set of challenges that required just as much attention, patience, and care.

The transition wasn't easy, and there were many moments when I felt frustrated, angry, and defeated.

But over time, I've learned to accept this new reality. My body will never function exactly as it did before, and I will always need to rely on medication to keep my hormones in balance. There are days when the fatigue is overwhelming, and I still struggle with weight gain and mood swings. But I've also found ways to manage these symptoms and adapt to life with hypothyroidism.

One of the key lessons I've learned is the importance of **self-compassion**. It's easy to be hard on yourself when your body isn't cooperating the way you want it to. I used to feel frustrated every time I gained weight, or when I couldn't keep up with the demands of daily life. But over time, I've realized that beating myself up only made things worse. Instead, I've learned to listen to my body, to give myself grace on the days when my energy is low, and to appreciate the small victories—like a day without joint pain, or the ability to go for a walk without feeling exhausted.

Mental health care became a vital part of my healing journey as well. Living with a chronic condition like hypothyroidism can take a toll on your emotional well-being, and for a long time, I tried to push through the depression and brain fog on my own. But I realized that I needed help. Seeking out therapy, talking about my struggles, and even journaling about my experiences helped me process the emotional weight I was carrying. It wasn't just about managing my physical symptoms—it was about taking care of my mind and soul, too.

One of the most profound changes has been the way I view **balance** in life. Before hypothyroidism, I was constantly pushing myself to do more—whether it was in my career, my relationships, or even just daily tasks. But living with an underactive thyroid forced me to slow down. I had no choice but to learn how to balance my energy levels and set boundaries for myself. It became clear that I couldn't do everything all at once, and that was okay. I began to prioritize rest, knowing that my body needed time to recharge, and I learned that taking things one step at a time was the key to managing my new normal.

Finding Strength in Vulnerability

Hypothyroidism brought challenges that I never anticipated, but it also taught me a great deal about my own resilience. For so long, I had viewed my health as something I could control—something that, with the right effort and mindset, I could manage on my own. But life after thyroidectomy taught me that true strength lies in acknowledging our vulnerabilities and asking for help when we need it.

There were many moments when I felt defeated—when the scale tipped higher, when my energy plummeted, when the pain in my feet made it difficult to walk. But in those moments, I found strength in reaching out to others, whether it was my doctors, my family, or friends who had experienced similar health struggles. I learned that living with a chronic illness doesn't mean you have to go it alone. In fact, it's the support of others that often helps us through the darkest times.

Community became an unexpected source of comfort. I began to connect with others who were going through similar thyroid journeys—people who had also undergone thyroidectomy, who were grappling with hypothyroidism, and who understood the emotional rollercoaster of managing a chronic condition. Through these connections, I realized that my struggles weren't unique, and that there were many others out there who could offer advice, share their stories, and provide encouragement. This sense of shared experience helped ease the isolation that so often accompanies chronic illness.

A New Perspective on Healing

Looking back on my journey from hyperthyroidism to hypothyroidism, I've come to understand that healing is not a linear process. It's not about reaching a point where everything is "fixed," but rather about finding ways to live in harmony with your body, even when it doesn't function the way it used to.

For a long time, I was focused on the idea of getting back to "normal"—the way my body used to feel before thyroid disease entered my life. But over time, I realized that this expectation was holding me back. I wasn't going to return to the person I was before, and that was okay. The journey of healing isn't about going backward—it's about moving forward with the knowledge and experience you've gained and finding a new kind of balance that works for you in the present moment.

Part of that new balance involved self-advocacy. After the surgery, I learned that I had to be my own advocate when it came to managing my thyroid hormone levels. There were times when my medication dosage didn't feel right, and I had to push for additional tests and adjustments. It wasn't always easy, doctors are busy, and thyroid disease can be tricky to manage. But I knew my body better than anyone else, and I had to trust myself to speak up when something felt off.

Over time, I've developed a greater understanding of how my body responds to medication, how different foods affect my energy levels, and how to manage stress in a way that doesn't exacerbate my symptoms. It's a constant learning process, but I've become more attuned to the signals my body sends me, and that awareness has been empowering.

Looking Forward: Embracing the Journey

The transition from hyperthyroidism to hypothyroidism has been a challenging and often overwhelming journey, but it has also been one of growth, resilience, and self-discovery. While the physical and emotional consequences of losing my thyroid are undeniable, I've found new ways to live a fulfilling life despite these challenges.

I've learned that managing a chronic condition requires more than just medication—it requires a holistic approach that includes **mental health care, self-compassion, lifestyle adjustments, and support from loved ones**. There is no quick fix for hypothyroidism, and there are days when the weight of it all feels heavy. But I've also learned that healing is about more than just feeling "better." It's about finding joy in the small victories, accepting where you are, and continuing to move forward, even when the path ahead is uncertain.

As I continue this journey, I know that there will be ups and downs. There will be days when the fatigue feels unbearable, when the weight gain is frustrating, and when the brain fog clouds my thoughts. But there will also be days when I feel strong, when I have energy, and when I can look back and see how far I've come.

Hypothyroidism may be a part of my life, but it doesn't define me. It's simply one chapter in a much larger story—one that's still unfolding. And through it all, I've learned that I am stronger, more resilient, and more capable than I ever imagined.

Chapter 5: Navigating the Healthcare System – Advocating for Myself

After my thyroidectomy, I thought I had finally reached a point of stability. The **100 mcg of levothyroxine** I was prescribed seemed to be doing the job, and my **TSH levels** were consistently within the "normal" range according to my lab results. At first, this was reassuring. I had been through the chaos of hyperthyroidism and was looking forward to moving past the constant fluctuations in my health. For a time, I believed that I was on the path to feeling "normal" again.

But as the months passed, I started to notice unsettling changes. My weight was steadily increasing, my energy levels were plummeting, and I was experiencing **brain fog** that made it difficult to concentrate or think clearly. Worst of all, I began to sink into **depression**, something I had never experienced before. The sadness was heavy, and I felt disconnected from myself. It was a dark period that made me question everything.

The Disconnect Between Lab Results and Symptoms

Despite how I was feeling, every blood test I took came back saying the same thing: my **TSH levels** were in the "normal" range. In the eyes of the medical system, I was perfectly fine. But how could I be fine when my body felt like it was shutting down? How could I be fine when I couldn't get through the day without feeling exhausted, when the weight kept piling on, and when I couldn't shake the fog that had settled over my mind? My doctor looked at my lab results and told me I was doing well, but nothing about my reality felt well.

It was deeply frustrating. I knew my body, and I knew something was wrong, but the medical system was telling me to accept that I was "normal" because my TSH numbers fell within a specific range. The

TSH test, I quickly learned, is often used as the primary diagnostic tool for thyroid health, but it doesn't always tell the full story. The test measures the level of thyroid-stimulating hormone in the blood, but it doesn't account for how the body is converting **T4 (levothyroxine)** into **T3**, the active hormone that regulates metabolism, energy, and mental clarity.

Through my own research, I discovered that many patients with hypothyroidism, like me, have trouble converting **T4** into **T3**. Instead of producing the active **T3 hormone**, my body was converting T4 into **reverse T3 (rT3)**—an inactive form of the hormone that blocks the effects of T3 and leads to the symptoms I was experiencing weight gain, fatigue, and mental fog. This revelation was both validating and frustrating—it explained why I was feeling so terrible despite my lab results, but it also left me wondering how I could fix it.

Frustration with the Pharmaceutical System

Once I learned about the role of **reverse T3**, I felt an overwhelming sense of frustration. Why wasn't this a part of the standard conversation between doctors and patients with thyroid issues? Why was the healthcare system so focused on the TSH test when it clearly didn't tell the whole story? I started to feel disillusioned with the **pharmaceutical system**, which seemed more interested in managing lab numbers than in addressing the actual well-being of patients.

It didn't make sense to me. The system seemed to be failing people like me—people whose TSH levels were "normal" but who were still experiencing debilitating symptoms. I couldn't help but question why it was so difficult to receive the right treatment for my body. The more I read about thyroid disorders, the more I realized I wasn't alone in this struggle. So many thyroid patients are stuck in this limbo, where their symptoms are dismissed simply because their lab results fall within a specific range.

I became increasingly frustrated with the rigidness of the pharmaceutical system. Why were there so many barriers to accessing treatments that could actually help patients feel better? It seemed like the system was more concerned with sticking to outdated protocols than with actually improving the quality of life for patients.

The Reverse T3 Problem: Seeking a Solution

Determined to find a solution, I requested a **reverse T3 (rT3)** test to confirm my suspicions. When the results came back, they confirmed what I had feared—my reverse T3 levels were high, which meant that my body wasn't converting T4 into the active T3 hormone it needed to function properly. This high level of reverse T3 was essentially blocking the positive effects of T3 and causing the symptoms that were making my life miserable.

Armed with this information, I returned to my doctor, hopeful that we could finally adjust my treatment plan. I had read about the benefits of adding **T3 (liothyronine)** to help counteract the high levels of reverse T3 and restore balance to my hormones. But when I asked my doctor about the possibility of adding T3 to my treatment, I was met with resistance. He refused to prescribe it, insisting that the **levothyroxine** I was already taking should be enough to manage my condition.

The Struggles with Healthcare Providers and the System

I was devastated. I had found a potential explanation for my symptoms, but I couldn't get the medication that might help me feel better. My doctor's refusal wasn't based on my individual case but rather on the strict **pharmaceutical regulations** surrounding T3 medication in Australia. T3 is considered a "last resort" treatment and is rarely prescribed, even when patients like me clearly need it. My doctor wasn't willing to deviate from the standard protocol, and there were legal and regulatory barriers that prevented him from doing so.

It felt like the system had failed me. Here I was, doing everything I could to advocate for my health, yet I was being denied the treatment that could potentially make a difference. I couldn't understand why it was so hard to access the medication I needed. Why was the system set up in such a way that it prioritized lab results over patient well-being? Why were doctors so reluctant to prescribe T3 when it was clear that levothyroxine alone wasn't enough?

This was a turning point for me. I realized that the healthcare system wasn't always going to have the answers, and I needed to start advocating for myself in a more assertive way.

Becoming My Own Advocate

I began to understand that if I wanted to improve my health, I couldn't rely solely on the traditional healthcare system. I had to **become my own advocate**. This wasn't just about finding the right medication—it was about standing up for my own needs, doing my research, and refusing to accept subpar care.

I threw myself into learning everything I could about thyroid health. I read medical journals, patient forums, and books on alternative treatments. I connected with online communities of thyroid patients, many of whom were experiencing the same struggles. It was empowering to see that I wasn't alone—there were others who had faced the same obstacles and had found ways to advocate for their own health.

One of the most important lessons I learned was that not all doctors are the same, and it's okay to seek out second opinions. I started searching for a doctor who might be more open to considering the bigger picture—someone who would look beyond the TSH numbers and listen to my symptoms. Unfortunately, in my case, I was unable to find a doctor in Australia who was willing to prescribe T3 due to the restrictive regulations.

This was a hard pill to swallow—quite literally. Despite my efforts, I couldn't access the medication I needed, and it felt like I had hit a dead end.

Living with Unanswered Questions

The inability to get my hands on **T3 medication** left me with more questions than answers. Why was I being denied a treatment that could potentially make a huge difference in my life? Why was the healthcare system so rigid when it came to thyroid treatment? The frustration I felt during this time was overwhelming. I had done everything right—I had researched, advocated, and pushed for the tests I needed, yet I was still being told that levothyroxine was my only option.

This experience made me question the larger **pharmaceutical system**. Why were patients like me being left to suffer simply because we didn't fit into a neat little box defined by lab results? Why was it so difficult to get access to treatments that could improve our lives? These questions lingered in my mind, and they fuelled a growing sense of disillusionment with the healthcare system. It wasn't enough to treat the numbers on a lab test—we needed doctors who were willing to treat the whole person.

The Power of Self-Advocacy Despite Setbacks

Although I wasn't able to access T3 medication, I didn't stop advocating for myself. I continued to explore other ways to manage my symptoms. I made adjustments to my lifestyle—focusing on **diet, stress management, and exercise**—to help mitigate the effects of hypothyroidism. I also learned the importance of mental health care, seeking support for the **depression** that had emerged as part of my condition.

What this journey taught me is that self-advocacy is about more than just medication. It's about learning to navigate a system that doesn't always have your best interests at heart. It's about understanding your body, educating yourself, and pushing back when something doesn't feel right. Even though I wasn't able to get the treatment I believed would help, I gained a sense of empowerment from knowing that I had done everything I could.

Moving Forward: Lessons in Resilience and Persistence

Looking back, I realize that my journey through the healthcare system wasn't just about managing hypothyroidism—it was about learning to stand up for myself and take control of my health. The frustration of being unable to access the medication I needed was real, but so was the resilience I built along the way. I learned that being informed and persistent is key to navigating a system that often prioritizes protocols over people.

Though I'm still on this journey, I now approach my health with a sense of empowerment. I've learned to ask questions, demand better care, and never stop searching for solutions. While I wasn't able to secure the treatment I had hoped for, I am better equipped to face whatever challenges come my way.

Chapter 6: Finding the Right Treatment Plan – What Worked for Me

After years of frustration and exhaustion from living with hypothyroidism, the medical system seemed to offer me no solutions. Levothyroxine, the standard medication prescribed after my thyroidectomy, simply wasn't working. Despite taking it regularly and having my TSH levels in the "normal" range, my body was telling a completely different story. I was experiencing constant **weight gain, brain fog, fatigue**, and a growing sense of **depression** that I couldn't shake. No matter how much I adjusted my lifestyle— healthy eating, regular exercise—nothing seemed to help. It became clear that my body wasn't converting **T4** (the hormone provided by levothyroxine) into **T3**, the active hormone needed to maintain a healthy metabolism and energy levels. The result was high levels of **reverse T3 (rT3)**, which explained my persistent symptoms.

Frustrated with the traditional treatments that weren't working, I knew I had to take matters into my own hands. I began to explore alternative solutions—looking for something that could help my body where levothyroxine was failing. After hours of research, reading, and digging through online forums, I stumbled upon something that would change my life: **natural desiccated thyroid (NDT)**, a medication derived from the thyroid glands of pigs, which closely resembles the hormones that a human thyroid naturally produces. Unlike synthetic options like levothyroxine, **NDT includes a full range of thyroid hormones—T4, T3, T2, T1, and calcitonin—** providing a more comprehensive approach to treating thyroid imbalances. This natural composition could potentially give my body the active **T3** it desperately needed, in addition to other important thyroid hormones that play a role in metabolism and overall health.

The Challenge of Accessing Natural Desiccated Thyroid (NDT)

Excited by the possibility of a more effective treatment, I began to look for ways to get my hands on **natural desiccated thyroid (NDT)**. However, I quickly realized that this was not going to be easy. In Australia, access to NDT is extremely limited, and it is not commonly prescribed by doctors. It's also not covered by the public health system, Medicare, which meant that even if I could find a doctor willing to prescribe it, the cost would be entirely out of pocket.

I scoured the internet, looking for clinics and doctors who might be open to prescribing NDT. I made countless phone calls, trying to find someone—anyone—who would help me. But time and time again, I was turned away. The few doctors who were familiar with NDT either weren't accepting new patients or were bound by restrictions that prevented them from prescribing it. Worse still, the cost of the medication was far beyond my financial means at the time. With the weight of my financial struggles on top of my health challenges, I felt like I was hitting brick walls at every turn.

For a while, I resigned myself to living with my symptoms. I couldn't afford NDT, and I couldn't find a doctor willing to prescribe it. So, I continued taking levothyroxine, hoping that somehow things would improve. But they didn't. My body continued to struggle. My feet would swell and ache after walking for even short periods, and I could barely stand in the shower for more than five minutes without pain. As someone who had been physically active and had trained in martial arts as a teenager, this decline was especially difficult for me to accept.

A Life-Changing Event: The Impact of Sepsis

In **January 2022**, my health took a turn for the worse in an unexpected way. I had my two wisdom teeth removed, and what followed was a nightmare. Unknown to me, I had developed a serious infection that led to **sepsis**, a life-threatening condition where the body's response to infection damages its own tissues and organs. For a month, the sepsis incubated silently, until I was rushed to the hospital in a delirious state, barely conscious and critically ill.

I spent over **three weeks** in the hospital recovering from the sepsis, but the damage had already been done. While I was thankful to have survived, sepsis wreaks havoc on the body's internal systems, and even though I was released from the hospital, I was no longer the person I had been before. My body felt weak, and my energy levels were lower than ever. The pain in my feet became unbearable. No matter how healthy I tried to eat or how carefully I exercised, I couldn't regain my strength.

On top of my hypothyroidism, sepsis had taken its toll on my circulatory system, leaving me feeling frustrated and broken. I knew in my heart that **levothyroxine** wasn't helping anymore, if it ever had at all. My symptoms were worsening, and I was becoming desperate for a solution.

The Determination to Try NDT

This time, I was determined to try **natural desiccated thyroid (NDT)**, no matter what it took. I knew from my research that NDT offered a more balanced approach to treating hypothyroidism by providing not just **T4**, but also **T3** and other essential thyroid hormones that the body needs to function properly.

With renewed determination, I resumed my search for a doctor who could prescribe **NDT**. After what felt like an endless search, I finally found a doctor—though in **Queensland**, a different state from where I live in **New South Wales**. This doctor, understanding my situation and desperation, was willing to consult with me over the phone. She agreed to prescribe NDT, and arranged for the medication to be compounded and sent to me from a pharmacy in Queensland.

Fortunately, by this time my financial situation had improved, and I was able to afford the cost of NDT, even though it wasn't subsidized by Medicare. When the medication finally arrived, I started taking it right away, and the effects were almost immediate. My **mood lifted**, my **energy returned**, and most importantly, the **pain in my feet** began to subside. I could stand in the shower for longer than five minutes without discomfort, and I could walk for more than 15 minutes without feeling like I needed to sit down. The **weight gain** that had plagued me for so long began to reverse, and for the first time in years, I felt like myself again. It was a revelation.

The Setback: A Costly Mistake

For six months, I took **natural desiccated thyroid** and felt incredible. My health improved in ways I hadn't experienced in years. I was so relieved that I had finally found something that worked. But then, a conversation with a well-meaning friend led me down a dangerous path. My friend recommended a book called "**Medical Healing: Thyroid Edition**," which suggested that even after a total thyroidectomy, the "soul" of the thyroid remains and that the thyroid could regenerate on its own. According to the book, it was possible to heal naturally through **detoxing** and **celery juice cleanses**.

Trusting the advice in the book, I made a decision that I would later deeply regret—I stopped taking NDT, believing that my thyroid could somehow regenerate and that I could live without medication. I threw myself into the **celery juice cleanse protocols**, and to be fair, I could see the benefits. I drank approximately 250ml of freshly juiced celery each morning on an empty stomach, making it a consistent part of my daily routine during that one-month celery juice cleanse period. The celery juice worked wonders on **cleaning my gut**, which I knew was crucial to overall health. A healthy gut plays an important role in ensuring a healthy body. I felt lighter and more energized in some ways, and I was grateful for the positive effects of the cleanse on my digestive system. However, despite the clear improvements in my gut health, it was a **big mistake** to go off the thyroid extract without consulting my doctor. Within just one month of going off NDT, my body spiralled. I gained **13 kilograms (approximately 29 pounds)**, and my body began to swell with water retention. My face puffed up, and I felt like I was slowing down visibly.

I realized too late that the book's advice didn't apply to me. My surgeon had removed **100% of my thyroid gland** during the thyroidectomy, and without a functioning thyroid, my body could not survive without hormone replacement. Without **T4** and **T3**, my metabolism was shutting down. If I had continued without treatment, I would have eventually entered a **myxoedema coma**, a life-threatening condition that occurs when hypothyroidism is left untreated.

I immediately called my doctor in Queensland, who was shocked to hear what I had done. She advised me to go back on NDT right away, and thankfully, within two months, I was able to lose the **13 kilograms** I had gained, and my symptoms began to improve again. This experience taught me a valuable lesson: not everything you read in a book is applicable to your specific situation, and it's important to consult with your healthcare provider before making any changes to your treatment plan.

A Devastating Blow: Losing Access to NDT

Just when I thought I had finally found a treatment that worked, I was dealt another blow. In **October 2023**, my doctor in Queensland sent me a letter informing me that due to restrictions placed on her by her medical insurance policy, she could no longer prescribe **natural desiccated thyroid**. This news was devastating. I had only a few days' worth of NDT left, and I had no idea where I would be able to find another doctor willing to prescribe it.

I went on a frantic quest, calling numerous clinics and integrated medicine practices, desperately trying to find someone who could help. Time after time, I was turned away. My frustration grew as I realized how **profit-driven** and **rigid** the medical system could be. It seemed like patient well-being was secondary to regulations and policies. At one point, I was so close to giving up. I even **broke down in tears** during an appointment with an integrated doctor who had initially given me hope but refused to prescribe NDT once we met face to face.

An Unexpected Help: Finding a New Doctor

Just when I thought I had exhausted all my options, a glimmer of hope appeared. One of the clinics I had called earlier phoned me back. They had a doctor who was willing to prescribe NDT, as long as I could provide proof that I had been prescribed it before. I couldn't believe it. This clinic was a **general practitioner's office**, which meant my consultation fees were affordable and subsidized by **Medicare**. And the best thing is, it is right where I live too. It felt like a miracle after so many setbacks. I was pleased to discover a compounding pharmacy right in my local shopping center, which was an added convenience.

I began taking **NDT** again, starting at **60 mcg** and gradually increasing to **95 mcg** before finally settling on **90 mcg**. I'm happy to report that my health has stabilized. At **5 feet 2 inches** tall, my weight is now steady at around **56 kilograms (123 pounds)**, and I finally feel a sense of balance that I hadn't experienced in years. My mood is stable, my energy is back, and my physical health has vastly improved.

A Cautionary Tale

Looking back on my journey, I've learned some hard but valuable lessons. It's easy to get swept up in the promises of alternative health solutions, especially when you're desperate for answers. But not everything applies to your unique situation, and it's essential to consult with professionals who understand your specific medical needs. Going off my medication based on the advice of a book was a mistake that nearly cost me my health. My experience serves as a reminder that while it's important to explore options, it's equally important to be careful and make informed decisions.

Conclusion

My journey through different medications, treatments, and alternatives has been long and filled with obstacles, but I finally found what works for me. **Natural desiccated thyroid** has been a game-changer, and while the road to getting it was difficult, the results have been worth it. My health, mood, and weight are now stable, and I feel like I've regained control of my life. If there's one thing I've learned, it's that the path to healing isn't always straightforward, but with persistence, research, and the right support, it's possible to find balance.

Chapter 7: Managing the Emotional Toll – Mental Health and Thyroid Disease

When we think about thyroid disease, we often focus on the physical symptoms—fatigue, weight gain or loss, changes in metabolism, and physical discomfort. But what is less talked about, and often underestimated, is the **psychological toll** that thyroid disorders take on a person's mental health. As someone who lived through the shift from **hyperthyroidism** to **hypothyroidism**, I experienced firsthand how these conditions affected not only my body but also my mind.

For years, I dealt with a barrage of emotional and mental health challenges, including **anxiety**, **depression**, and overwhelming **stress**. Thyroid disease can alter brain chemistry, leading to shifts in mood, motivation, and overall mental well-being. It's a part of the disease that isn't always visible to others, but it's one that deeply impacts the daily lives of those suffering from thyroid disorders. What I've come to understand through my journey is that **healing from thyroid disease is not just about finding the right medication**—it's about **managing life's stresses** and navigating the emotional landscape that comes with living with a chronic illness.

Our health is directly tied to our emotional and mental conditions. When our lives are filled with stress, uncertainty, and emotional upheaval, it can significantly affect our physical health, and for those of us with thyroid disorders, the impact can be even greater. Learning to manage not only the physical symptoms of thyroid disease but also the emotional challenges is crucial to finding true balance and healing.

The Psychological Effects of Thyroid Disorders

The connection between thyroid health and mental health is undeniable. The thyroid gland plays a key role in regulating hormones that affect nearly every part of the body, including the brain. When thyroid hormone levels are too high or too low, it can result in a range of psychological symptoms that can feel confusing and overwhelming. During my experience with **hyperthyroidism**, I was often filled with **anxiety**. My mind raced alongside my heart, and I struggled to find any sense of calm or peace. The rapid-fire thoughts, restlessness, and irritability left me feeling out of control, and I often found myself snapping at loved ones over the smallest things.

But the shift to **hypothyroidism** after my thyroidectomy brought an entirely different set of mental health challenges. Instead of feeling wired and anxious, I was suddenly overwhelmed with feelings of sadness and despair. It wasn't just the **fatigue** or the **weight gain** that weighed on me—there was a deep sense of **hopelessness** that crept in, a feeling that no matter what I did, I couldn't get my life back on track. This **depression** was unlike anything I had ever experienced before, and it was made even more isolating by the fact that from the outside, no one could see what I was going through.

The **brain fog** that accompanied hypothyroidism was one of the most frustrating symptoms. It felt like my mind was clouded, like I was walking through life in a haze. Tasks that used to be easy became difficult, and I constantly felt as though I was forgetting something or couldn't concentrate. This fog, combined with the depression, made even the simplest things feel overwhelming. My self-esteem took a major hit, as I found it harder and harder to recognize myself. The person I had once been—sharp, energetic, and capable—felt lost beneath the weight of my thyroid disease.

Managing Stress, Anxiety, and Depression

Dealing with these psychological symptoms wasn't easy. In fact, it often felt like I was in a constant battle to reclaim my mental health. One of the first steps I took was recognizing that stress, anxiety, and **depression** were not just side effects of life—they were directly tied to my thyroid condition. This acknowledgment helped me approach my mental health in a new way, understanding that managing my thyroid was as much about supporting my mind as it was about healing my body.

One of the most important lessons I learned was that **managing life's stressors** was a critical part of managing my thyroid condition. Stress has a profound impact on thyroid function, and in my case, I noticed that during periods of high stress, my symptoms would intensify. Whether it was the racing thoughts of hyperthyroidism or the crushing fatigue and hopelessness of hypothyroidism, stress only made everything worse. I had to learn that taking care of my emotional well-being wasn't a luxury—it was a necessity for my overall health.

Managing stress became a central focus for me. I began to explore ways to **manage anxiety** and create a sense of calm in my day-to-day routine. One of the most effective tools for me was **mindful breathing and meditation**. At first, it was difficult to sit still with my racing thoughts, but over time, I found that even just a few minutes of deep breathing could help centre me and ease the tension that seemed to live in my body. It wasn't a cure, but it gave me the space to slow down, both physically and mentally.

I also found that staying active—though difficult at times— played a significant role in managing my mood. During hyperthyroidism, intense exercise wasn't an option, but I found that **low-impact activities** like walking or yoga helped release nervous energy and calm my mind. When hypothyroidism took over, and I struggled with fatigue, even a short walk around the neighborhood helped lift my spirits. These small acts of movement not only helped with my physical health but also improved my emotional state.

Coping Strategies for Emotional Well-Being

Over time, I developed several strategies that helped me maintain my emotional well-being, even during the most difficult days. These strategies became just as important as finding the right medication, because healing from thyroid disease is about more than just taking a pill—it's about creating an environment where both the body and mind can thrive.

1. **Seeking Professional Support:** Although I personally didn't seek professional help, I strongly recommend that other patients consider it if they feel the need. Speaking to a therapist or counsellor can be incredibly beneficial in managing the overwhelming feelings of anxiety, depression, and confusion that often accompany thyroid disorders. Having someone to talk to, who can help you reframe your thoughts and provide clarity, may offer a significant boost to emotional recovery and well-being.

2. **Establishing a Routine**: Creating a **daily routine** gave me a sense of control over my life when everything felt chaotic. Hypothyroidism often left me feeling disorganized and scattered, with the **brain fog** making it difficult to complete tasks. By setting small, achievable goals each day—whether it was taking a walk, preparing a healthy meal, or setting aside time for rest—I was able to regain some structure and reduce the anxiety that came from feeling like I was losing control.

3. **Building a Support System**: Thyroid disease can feel incredibly isolating, especially when others around you can't see what you're experiencing. I made an effort to connect with others who were also dealing with thyroid conditions, whether through online forums or support groups. Knowing that there were others who understood what I was going through provided me with

comfort and reminded me that I wasn't alone in this struggle.

4. **Self-Compassion**: One of the hardest but most necessary things I learned was to be **compassionate with myself**. When I first began experiencing the mental health effects of thyroid disease, I was hard on myself, feeling guilty for being less productive, for gaining weight, or for needing more rest. But over time, I learned to be gentler with myself. I started to understand that this wasn't a failure on my part—this was a condition I was managing, and it was okay to take things slower. Practicing self-compassion helped me rebuild my self-esteem and allowed me to move through the challenges with more patience and kindness toward myself.

5. **Diet and Nutrition**: **Nutrition** played a critical role in supporting my mental health. I focused on a diet rich in whole foods—plenty of fruits, vegetables, lean proteins, and healthy fats—that helped support my thyroid function and overall well-being. Eating nutrient-dense foods gave me the energy I needed to tackle the day and helped lift my mood. I also made sure to stay hydrated and avoid processed foods, which only seemed to exacerbate my symptoms.

6. **Sharing My Experience:** Instead of journaling and reflecting privately, I felt an overwhelming urge to put my experience out there in the hopes of helping others going through the same struggles. Writing about my journey became less about self-reflection and more about providing guidance and support to others. By sharing my story, I could process my emotions while also offering a lifeline to those who, like me, felt lost in the complexities of thyroid disease. Knowing that my experiences could benefit others gave me a sense of purpose and helped me find hope, even during the darker moments.

Healing is Holistic

Through my journey, I've come to realize that **healing from thyroid disease isn't just about finding the right medication**—it's about **managing life's stresses**, cultivating emotional resilience, and creating an environment where your body and mind can heal together. Thyroid disease affects every aspect of your being, and true healing requires a holistic approach that addresses both the physical and emotional toll.

As I've learned to manage my thyroid condition, I've also learned to **manage my life** in new ways. I've had to become more mindful of stress and its impact on my health. I've had to create routines that support my well-being, practice self-compassion, and seek out support when I need it. Each of these practices has been vital to my healing process, and they have helped me move forward with a sense of empowerment and balance.

Chapter 8: Diet, Lifestyle, and Supplements for Thyroid Health

Thyroid disorders are complex and require a multifaceted approach to management. Beyond medication, **diet, lifestyle changes, and supplements** play a crucial role in supporting thyroid health and improving overall well-being. Whether you're dealing with **hyperthyroidism** (an overactive thyroid) or **hypothyroidism** (an underactive thyroid), making targeted adjustments to your diet, incorporating the right supplements, and adopting a balanced lifestyle can significantly improve your quality of life.

When I was struggling with hypothyroidism, I learned that even small changes could lead to significant improvements over time. Finding balance wasn't an overnight success—it required persistence and a willingness to make ongoing adjustments to my lifestyle. Whether you're managing **hyperthyroidism** or **hypothyroidism**, I've learned that it's possible to regain control of your health by listening to your body, making mindful choices, and staying consistent.

A Holistic Approach to Thyroid Wellness

Thyroid disorders don't exist in isolation. The thyroid gland, often referred to as the "master gland" of metabolism, affects nearly every system in the body—digestion, energy production, mental clarity, sleep, and emotional stability. Thus, when the thyroid is out of balance, it's crucial to focus on **holistic healing**—a full-body, full-mind approach that involves nourishing yourself physically, mentally, and emotionally.

For many people, especially those who suffer from **hypothyroidism**, the road to recovery can feel like an uphill battle.

You may experience **unexplained weight gain, sluggishness, hair loss**, and **depression**. It's a tough reality to face when your own body feels like it's betraying you. Meanwhile, those dealing with **hyperthyroidism** may feel trapped in a constant state of **overdrive**, with **anxiety, heart palpitations**, and **insomnia** becoming unwelcome companions. In both cases, it's easy to feel overwhelmed, but it's important to remember that taking small, consistent steps can gradually restore balance and improve your quality of life.

One of the most important lessons I've learned is that **healing from thyroid disease** is not just about finding the right medication. It's about managing your entire life—the food you eat, how you handle stress, your exercise routine, and even how you emotionally respond to challenges. Each of these factors has a direct impact on your thyroid and overall health. **Your body and mind are interconnected** and caring for one means caring for the other.

Effective Supplements for Thyroid Health

Supplements can provide a powerful boost to thyroid function when combined with the right diet and lifestyle adjustments. Whether you're dealing with an underactive or overactive thyroid, certain vitamins, minerals, and herbs can help fill in the gaps that medications alone may not address. However, supplements are not a magic cure—they work best when they complement a balanced diet and healthy lifestyle.

Here are some highly reviewed supplements that can support thyroid health, based on expert advice and feedback from thyroid patients around the world:

Supplements for Hyperthyroidism

If you have **hyperthyroidism**, supporting your body as it navigates an overproduction of thyroid hormones is critical. The goal is to calm the thyroid and provide essential nutrients to help manage the strain on your body's systems.

1. **L-Carnitine**: Studies suggest that **L-carnitine** may help alleviate some of the hyperthyroid symptoms by inhibiting the uptake of thyroid hormones into the cells. Carnitine is particularly useful in managing **muscle weakness** and **rapid heartbeat**—two common symptoms of hyperthyroidism.

2. **Magnesium**: **Magnesium** is essential for hundreds of bodily functions, and it is especially important for those with hyperthyroidism, as it can help relax muscles and regulate heart function. Taking **magnesium citrate** or **magnesium glycinate** can relieve **muscle cramps, tension**, and **heart palpitations**. Magnesium also helps manage **insomnia** and **anxiety**, two common complaints of hyperthyroid patients.

3. **Omega-3 Fatty Acids: Fish oil supplements** rich in **EPA and DHA** can help reduce the inflammation often present in those with hyperthyroidism. Omega-3s also support heart health, which is crucial for those whose thyroid has overworked the cardiovascular system.

4. **Vitamin D**: **Hyperthyroidism** can lead to a loss in **bone density** over time. Taking **Vitamin D3** can help prevent bone loss, especially in patients who are at risk of **osteoporosis**. Combining it with **calcium** supplements can further protect against the weakening of bones.

5. **Melatonin**: Hyperthyroidism often leads to **insomnia** due to an overactive thyroid. **Melatonin supplements** can help regulate the sleep-wake cycle, allowing for better rest and recovery.

Supplements for Hypothyroidism

For those with **hypothyroidism**, the focus shifts to boosting thyroid hormone production and supporting energy levels. Hypothyroidism often leads to **fatigue, depression**, and **weight gain**, so supplements that target these symptoms can make a significant difference.

1. **Selenium**: As one of the most important nutrients for thyroid health, **selenium** is necessary for converting T4 into the active T3 hormone. Research has shown that selenium supplementation can reduce the autoimmune activity in **Hashimoto's thyroiditis** and improve **thyroid hormone conversion**. Patients who take selenium often report better energy levels, improved **mood**, and more stable **weight management**.

2. **Ashwagandha**: This **adaptogenic herb** has been praised for its ability to **balance thyroid hormones** and reduce symptoms of hypothyroidism. Ashwagandha helps by supporting the **adrenal glands**, which are often overworked in hypothyroidism. It's also noted for its ability to combat **fatigue** and improve **mental clarity**.

3. **Vitamin B Complex**: A deficiency in **B vitamins**, particularly **B12** and **B6**, is common in people with hypothyroidism. Supplementing with a **B-complex** can help improve **energy levels**, enhance **cognitive function**, and support **metabolism**. Many patients have noticed a reduction in **brain fog** and improved **mental clarity** after consistent B-complex supplementation.

4. **Probiotics**: The connection between gut health and thyroid function cannot be ignored. Taking a **high-quality probiotic supplement** can improve digestion, reduce **constipation**, and support immune function, all of which are critical in hypothyroidism. Probiotics also help improve nutrient absorption, which is often impaired in thyroid conditions.

5. **Iodine (with caution)**: For patients with non-autoimmune hypothyroidism, iodine can be beneficial in promoting thyroid hormone production. However, **iodine** supplementation must be approached carefully, especially for those with **Hashimoto's**, as excess iodine can exacerbate autoimmune attacks on the thyroid. Always consult with a healthcare professional before introducing iodine into your regimen.

Diet and Nutrition: Supporting Thyroid Health Through Food

Diet plays a central role in supporting thyroid health. Whether you're trying to calm an overactive thyroid or stimulate an underactive one, the foods you consume can either support or hinder your progress. Whole foods, rich in essential nutrients, provide the foundation for thyroid health and overall well-being.

Foods to Support Hyperthyroidism

- **Cruciferous Vegetables**: **Broccoli**, **cauliflower**, **kale**, and other cruciferous vegetables can help reduce thyroid hormone production. Try to include these vegetables regularly in your diet, particularly when lightly cooked, as cooking reduces their goitrogenic effects.
- **Antioxidant-Rich Foods**: Hyperthyroidism can increase oxidative stress in the body. To counteract this, focus on foods high in antioxidants, such as **berries**, **green tea**, and **dark leafy greens**. These help to neutralize free radicals and reduce inflammation.
- **Healthy Fats**: Incorporate **avocados**, **olive oil**, and **coconut oil** into your diet to support hormone regulation and improve energy levels. These healthy fats can also help keep your heart healthy, which is crucial in hyperthyroidism.
- **Proteins**: Since hyperthyroidism accelerates muscle breakdown, it's important to include adequate **protein** in your diet. Focus on lean sources like **chicken**, **turkey**, **beans**, and **legumes** to maintain muscle mass and support energy levels.

Foods to Support Hypothyroidism

- **Sea Vegetables**: **Seaweed** is one of the best sources of iodine for supporting thyroid function. Incorporate small amounts of

nori, **wakame**, or **dulse** into your diet if your iodine levels are low.

- **Selenium-Rich Foods**: As with supplements, consuming foods high in selenium, such as **Brazil nuts**, **sunflower seeds**, and **tuna**, can improve thyroid function.

- **Fiber-Rich Foods**: Since hypothyroidism often leads to **constipation**, focus on foods that promote healthy digestion, such as **oats**, **chia seeds**, **berries**, and **leafy greens**. These help keep your digestive system regular.

- **Iron-Rich Foods**: **Iron deficiency** is common in hypothyroidism, which can exacerbate fatigue and brain fog. Add **lentils**, **red meat**, **spinach**, and **fortified cereals** to ensure you're getting enough iron.

Exercise and Lifestyle for Thyroid Health

Exercise is a key component of thyroid health, but it's essential to tailor your activity to your specific condition. Whether you're dealing with hyperthyroidism or hypothyroidism, maintaining an **active lifestyle** can greatly support both physical and emotional health.

Exercise for Hyperthyroidism

Because hyperthyroidism can cause **muscle weakness** and **fatigue**, it's important to engage in **low-impact** and **gentle exercises**. Activities like **yoga**, **walking**, and **stretching** are beneficial for maintaining muscle tone without overstimulating the body.

- **Yoga and Meditation**: Incorporating **yoga** into your routine can help reduce stress and balance the nervous system, which is often overstimulated in hyperthyroidism. Yoga's emphasis on breathing also helps reduce anxiety and improves mental clarity.

- **Light Weight Training**: **Resistance exercises** using

light weights or body weight can help maintain muscle mass and improve overall strength without putting too much strain on your body.

Exercise for Hypothyroidism

Hypothyroidism often leads to **weight gain** and **fatigue**, so exercise can help by boosting metabolism and improving energy levels. However, starting slow is key, especially when energy levels are low.

- **Cardiovascular Exercise**: Low-impact cardiovascular exercises like **walking**, **swimming**, and **cycling** can help burn calories and stimulate the metabolism. Aim for **30 minutes of movement a day**, but listen to your body and adjust as needed.
- **Strength Training**: Building **muscle mass** is essential in hypothyroidism, as muscle helps increase metabolic rate. Incorporate **weight training** exercises, such as squats, lunges, and resistance band exercises, into your weekly routine.
- **Stretching and Mobility**: Since hypothyroidism can cause joint pain and stiffness, regular **stretching** and **mobility exercises** can help improve flexibility and reduce discomfort.

Practical Wellness Tips for Thyroid Health

In addition to diet, supplements, and exercise, there are a few other key practices that can help support your thyroid and overall well-being:

1. **Stay Hydrated**: Drinking enough water is critical for maintaining **metabolism** and **digestion**, especially in hypothyroidism. Aim to drink at least **2-3 liters of water** per day.
2. **Manage Stress**: Chronic stress can wreak havoc on thyroid

function, so incorporating **stress-reduction techniques** like meditation, deep breathing, or spending time in nature can help balance hormones and improve overall health.

3. **Get Enough Sleep**: Both hyperthyroidism and hypothyroidism can disrupt sleep patterns. Prioritize getting **7-8 hours of quality sleep** per night to help your body recover and maintain balance.

4. **Monitor Your Thyroid Levels**: Regular check-ups with your doctor are essential for monitoring your thyroid hormone levels. This helps ensure that your treatment plan is effective and allows for adjustments as needed.

5. **Stay Consistent**: Whether it's your diet, supplements, or exercise routine, consistency is key. Small, consistent changes lead to long-term improvement in your thyroid health and overall well-being.

Conclusion

Managing thyroid health is about far more than just finding the right medication. While medication can be a crucial component of treatment, true healing requires a **holistic approach** that nurtures both your thyroid and your entire body. The thyroid, small though it may be, plays an essential role in your overall health, affecting everything from your metabolism and energy levels to your mood and mental clarity. This is why supporting it requires attention to every aspect of your life—diet, supplements, exercise, and stress management all play significant roles in your recovery and long-term well-being.

By focusing on a **nutrient-dense diet**, you give your body the building blocks it needs to function optimally. The right foods can help calm an overactive thyroid or boost an underactive one, and they provide the energy and nourishment your body needs to handle everyday stress. Incorporating **targeted supplements** that fill nutritional gaps and address your unique needs ensures that your thyroid and overall health remain well-supported. Supplements like selenium, magnesium, and omega-3 fatty acids can significantly improve thyroid function and help manage symptoms more effectively when used as part of a comprehensive plan.

However, it's not just about what you consume. Staying **physically active** plays a vital role in boosting your energy levels, managing weight, and improving mood—whether you are battling the exhaustion of hypothyroidism or the overdrive of hyperthyroidism. It's important to find an exercise routine that fits your energy levels and supports your specific condition, ensuring that your body is moving in a way that feels good without causing unnecessary strain.

Perhaps one of the most underrated, yet crucial, components of thyroid health is **stress management**. Chronic stress can be a major trigger for thyroid imbalances and can worsen symptoms. It's essential to develop strategies that help you manage life's stressors, whether through meditation, yoga, breathing exercises, or simply finding time to unwind and relax. Stress has a profound impact on the thyroid, and learning to manage it is one of the most empowering steps you can take for your health.

It's also important to recognize that **healing from thyroid disease is a journey**—one that requires patience, persistence, and self-compassion. There may be ups and downs along the way, and not every day will feel like progress, but each small step you take brings you closer to reclaiming your health. Whether it's incorporating a new supplement, making small adjustments to your diet, or finding a new way to manage stress, every positive change counts. The process of healing is gradual, and the more you listen to your body, the more attuned you become to what it needs to thrive.

Thyroid disorders, whether hyperthyroidism or hypothyroidism, can feel overwhelming at times. They affect your physical health, your mental clarity, and even your emotional well-being. But through a balanced, consistent approach, it is possible to regain control. The journey to wellness is deeply personal, and finding what works best for your body may take time. But each action you take—whether it's incorporating healthier foods, staying active, or finding moments of calm amidst the stress—brings you closer to feeling like yourself again.

Lastly, it's essential to be **patient with yourself** throughout this process. Healing is rarely linear, and setbacks are a natural part of the journey. Remember to celebrate small victories along the way— whether it's a boost in energy, a clearer mind, or even just feeling more grounded and connected to your body. These moments of progress, no matter how small, are signs that you're moving in the right direction.

In the end, managing thyroid health is about learning to take care of your whole self. It's about recognizing the interconnectedness of your body and mind, and understanding that supporting your thyroid means supporting your entire being. With the right balance of diet, supplements, exercise, and stress management, you can make a meaningful difference in how you feel, and most importantly, you can reclaim your vitality, your energy, and your well-being.

Remember, healing from thyroid disease is a journey, not a destination. Each step forward is a victory, and with dedication, patience, and the right support, you will find your way to renewed health and balance.

Lastly, it's essential to be patient with yourself throughout this process. Healing is rarely linear, and setbacks are a natural part of the journey. Remember to celebrate small victories along the way— whether it's a boost in energy, a clearer mind, or even just feeling more grounded and connected to your body. These moments of progress, no matter how small, are signs that you're moving in the right direction.

In the end, managing thyroid health is about learning to take care of your whole self. It's about recognizing the interconnectedness of your body and mind, and understanding that supporting your thyroid means supporting your entire being. With the right balance of diet, supplements, exercise, and stress management, you can make a meaningful difference in how you feel, and most importantly, you can reclaim your vitality, your energy, and your well-being.

Remember, healing from thyroid disease is a journey, not a destination. Each step forward is a victory, and with dedication, patience, and the right support, you will find your way to renewed health and balance.

Chapter 9: Lessons Learned – What I Wish I Knew Earlier

The road through thyroid disease is full of unexpected twists and turns. Along my journey, I've experienced both extremes—going from hyperthyroidism to hypothyroidism after undergoing a total thyroidectomy. These experiences have taught me valuable lessons that I wish I had known earlier, not just about the thyroid itself but about how to approach healing holistically, how to navigate the medical system, and how important it is to advocate for yourself every step of the way.

When I was first diagnosed with hyperthyroidism, I had no idea what was in store for me. At the time, I was focused on finding a quick solution to my symptoms—the racing heart, anxiety, and the feeling that my body was constantly in overdrive. I was a new mother, juggling a difficult marriage, work, and studies, and the thought of living with these exhausting symptoms was unbearable. What I didn't realize back then was that healing from thyroid disease is not a one-size-fits-all journey, and the decisions we make—particularly when it comes to treatment—can have lifelong consequences.

If you're reading this as someone who is newly diagnosed, or perhaps someone who has been struggling with their thyroid condition for a while, I want to share some of the key lessons I've learned through my experience. These lessons are the things I wish I had known earlier, and they have shaped the way I approach my health today.

1. A Holistic Approach to Healing: What I Would Have Done Differently

One of the biggest things I've come to realize is that healing from thyroid disease is **about much more than just medication**. Looking back, I wish I had taken a more **holistic approach** to my hyperthyroidism instead of rushing toward what I thought was a permanent fix—**total thyroidectomy**. At the time, I was desperate for relief from the constant physical and emotional strain of my overactive thyroid. But now I understand that my thyroidectomy was not the only solution, and I wish I had explored **natural and alternative** methods before making such a drastic decision.

If I were still managing hyperthyroidism today, I would have given myself the time and space to look inward and make changes to how I dealt with stress. For me, stress was a major trigger that made my symptoms worse. And, like many of us, I found myself in situations where stress was unavoidable, particularly in a difficult marriage. But I've learned over time that **walking away from toxic or stressful environments** is not just an emotional decision—it's a necessary step in preserving your health. No amount of medication can undo the damage caused by constant stress.

Beyond managing stress, I would have focused on cleansing my gut and adjusting my diet and lifestyle to better support my thyroid health. I learned much later in my journey that gut health plays a crucial role in thyroid function. A diet rich in **anti-inflammatory foods, probiotics, and nutrient-dense meals** could have been the foundation for a more natural recovery. Had I incorporated meditation, calmness practices, and supplements that supported thyroid health, I believe I could have managed my hyperthyroid symptoms more effectively.

Staying on antithyroid medication for a longer period would have also given me the time I needed to explore these holistic options. Instead, I rushed into the idea of surgery because I thought it was the only solution. Looking back, I now know that unless surgery is absolutely medically necessary, it's worth taking the time to see if your thyroid can heal naturally with the right lifestyle changes. **Once your thyroid is gone, it's gone**—there's no turning back after a total thyroidectomy.

2. The Consequences of Total Thyroidectomy: From One Extreme to Another

One of the hardest lessons I learned was that a **total thyroidectomy** doesn't necessarily "fix" everything—it just shifts the problem to the opposite end of the spectrum. I went from dealing with an overactive thyroid that made me feel like my body was always on fast-forward, to struggling with an underactive thyroid that made everything feel slow and heavy.

Hypothyroidism brought on a whole new set of challenges. Instead of anxiety and restlessness, I now faced **fatigue, weight gain**, and a deep sense of **mental fog**. Tasks that had once felt easy now required tremendous effort. I went from one extreme—feeling wired and overstimulated all the time—to another, where I felt sluggish, unmotivated, and mentally unclear. The weight gain was especially frustrating, as no matter what I tried, it seemed impossible to keep it off.

But perhaps one of the most surprising and heartbreaking consequences of my surgery was how it impacted my **fertility**. After the thyroidectomy, I learned that my chances of getting pregnant had been significantly reduced. This was a devastating realization because I had never fully understood the long-term effects of thyroid surgery on reproductive health. My thyroidectomy didn't just impact my metabolism—it affected my body in ways I hadn't anticipated, and this is something I wish more people were aware of before making such a life-changing decision.

If you're considering a thyroidectomy, my advice is to be fully informed about what comes next. Removing your thyroid may resolve some issues, but it creates new ones. Once you are hypothyroid, you'll be on **hormone replacement** therapy for the rest of your life, and managing hypothyroidism can be just as challenging as managing hyperthyroidism. I wish I had been told that transitioning to hypothyroidism would bring its own set of difficulties, and that surgery isn't always the clear-cut solution it seems to be.

3. The Pharmaceutical System: A Hard Lesson in Self-Advocacy

One of the most eye-opening experiences of my thyroid journey was realizing how the **pharmaceutical system** operates—and it's not always in the patient's best interest. When I was first prescribed **levothyroxine** after my surgery, I assumed it was the best and only option for managing my hypothyroidism. But as the months went by, I began to experience troubling symptoms—**weight gain**, **brain fog**, and even **depression**, things I had never dealt with before. Despite my **TSH levels** being within the "normal" range, I felt anything but normal. This disconnect between lab results and how I actually felt was a turning point for me. It made me question the entire system I had been relying on.

After doing some research, I discovered that there was an alternative—**natural desiccated thyroid (NDT)**. NDT, derived from pig thyroid glands, contains not only **T4**, but also **T3, T2, T1**, and **calcitonin**, making it a more complete and holistic treatment for hypothyroidism. It had been used for decades before synthetic **T4-only medications** like levothyroxine were introduced. What shocked me was that **NDT** had fallen out of favor not because it was less effective, but because **T4-only medications could be patented**. Since natural substances like desiccated thyroid extract can't be patented, the pharmaceutical industry pushed synthetic alternatives for profit.

Learning this was devastating. Here I was, struggling with the side effects of levothyroxine, when a more natural, effective option existed all along—but it was being restricted. The **medical and pharmaceutical industries** are profit-driven, and they often prioritize treatments that generate revenue over those that may truly benefit patients. I've since learned that I'm not alone in this. Many people with hypothyroidism struggle to access **NDT**, even though it can be life-changing for those whose bodies don't convert **T4** to **T3** efficiently.

Had I known about **NDT** earlier, I would have advocated for it from the start. But it took me a long time to understand that **self-advocacy** is essential. You have to be willing to ask questions, challenge the status quo, and seek out second opinions. Doctors don't always have the full picture, and the pharmaceutical system is designed to push certain treatments over others. Don't be afraid to fight for the treatment that feels right for you.

4. Advice for Newly Diagnosed Patients: You Have More Power Than You Think

If you've recently been diagnosed with a thyroid disorder, I know how overwhelming it can feel. The symptoms, the doctor's visits, the tests—it can make you feel like you've lost control of your own body. But I'm here to tell you that you have more power than you think. **Patience**, **persistence**, and **self-advocacy** are your best tools in this journey.

Here are a few things I wish I had known earlier:

• **Explore All Your Options**: Don't rush into any major decisions about surgery or medication. Take the time to explore all of your options, including **holistic approaches** and **alternative treatments**. It's important to understand that there are multiple paths to healing.

• **Trust Your Body**: You know your body better than anyone. If something doesn't feel right, whether it's a medication or a doctor's advice, don't be afraid to question it. If you feel like your symptoms aren't improving, even if your lab results are "normal," trust yourself and seek further opinions.

- **Be Informed**: Knowledge is power. Take the time to learn about your thyroid condition, the available treatments, and the latest research. Don't rely solely on what your doctor tells you. The more informed you are, the better equipped you'll be to make decisions that support your health.

- **Find the Right Doctor**: Not every doctor will be a good fit for you. It's important to find a healthcare provider who listens to you, respects your concerns, and is open to exploring different treatment options. A doctor who understands that **thyroid health is complex** will make all the difference.

5. Persistence and Self-Advocacy: Never Stop Fighting for Your Health

Throughout my thyroid journey, I've learned that **healing is not a straight line**. There are setbacks, moments of frustration, and times when you feel like giving up. But persistence is key. Whether it's advocating for the right medication, seeking out alternative treatments, or making small lifestyle changes, each step forward brings you closer to regaining control of your health.

You have to keep pushing for the treatment that works for you. Be persistent with your doctors, don't settle for answers that don't feel right, and continue to advocate for your health. It's easy to feel lost in a system that sometimes prioritizes profit over well-being, but you have the power to take charge of your journey.

Conclusion

The lessons I've learned on this journey are ones I wish I could have known earlier, but they've shaped the way I approach my health now. My hope is that by sharing these insights, I can help others navigate their thyroid journey with greater clarity and confidence.

Remember, your health is your most valuable asset, and it's worth fighting for. **Stay informed, be persistent, and always advocate for what's best for you.** With the right approach, you can reclaim your life from thyroid disease and move forward feeling empowered, healthy, and whole.

Chapter 10: My Personal Routine for Managing Underactive Thyroid

Living with hypothyroidism has been a journey of constant learning, adjustment, and self-discipline. After my total thyroidectomy, I quickly realized that the key to managing my condition effectively would be through developing a personal routine that supported my overall well-being. It hasn't always been easy, but over time, I've discovered what works best for my body, and I've committed myself to making small but significant changes that help me feel healthier, stronger, and more balanced.

I want to share with you what my daily routine looks like in the hopes that it might inspire you to create your own. Keep in mind that every person is different, and what works for me might not work exactly the same way for you, but I believe that developing a routine, listening to your body, and being consistent are universal principles that can benefit anyone dealing with an underactive thyroid.

1. Morning Ritual: Starting the Day Right

The first thing I do every morning is take my **thyroid extract**. It's the very first thing I put into my body when I wake up, and I make sure to take it at the **same time** every day. I've found that maintaining this consistency has made a huge difference in how my body processes the medication. In fact, one of my close friends, who also had a total thyroidectomy, struggled with getting pregnant despite being young and otherwise healthy. Her doctor recommended that she take her thyroid hormone at the exact same time every morning, and after about a year of doing so, she was able to conceive. This experience reinforced the importance of timing and routine in managing my own thyroid health.

After taking my thyroid extract, I usually begin getting ready for the day, whether it's for work or other activities. **Half an hour or an hour later after I took my thyroid extract**, I drink my morning **elixir**—a simple but powerful drink that I believe has done wonders for my metabolism and overall well-being. It's a warm cup of water with the juice from half a lemon squeezed into it, a pinch of **natural unrefined salt** (like Celtic salt), and occasionally, a teaspoon of **raw sugarcane sugar**. Sometimes, I also add a pinch of **cayenne pepper** for an extra kick. This drink has become an integral part of my morning routine because it helps with my **blood circulation**, boosts my **metabolism**, and most importantly, supports my **liver health**.

As you may know, the liver is our body's main **detoxifying organ**, and keeping it functioning optimally is crucial, especially for those with thyroid issues. The liver plays a significant role in the conversion of thyroid hormones, so supporting its health is essential for maintaining balanced thyroid function. This warm drink is like a gentle tonic that prepares my body for the day ahead.

2. Embracing Intermittent Fasting

For the past year, I've been practicing **intermittent fasting**, and it has made a noticeable difference in how I manage my weight and energy levels. My approach is simple—I aim to finish my **last meal before 7 pm**, and then I refrain from eating until **10:30 am** the next morning. During this fasting window, I allow myself to have my thyroid extract, my morning drink, and water.

Intermittent fasting works well for me because it gives my digestive system a break, allowing my body to focus on other vital functions, like healing and repair. Around **10:30 am**, I'll break my fast with something light, like an apple or a banana. I find that easing into food after fasting helps keep my energy stable throughout the day. Since my work in the office doesn't require intense physical activity, intermittent fasting fits naturally into my routine without leaving me feeling overly hungry or fatigued. Of course, this practice may not work for everyone, so it's important to listen to your body and adjust accordingly.

3. Balanced, Moderate Eating

When it comes to meals, I don't follow a rigid diet, but I focus on **moderation** and **balance**. I generally cook and eat at home, and my diet includes a variety of **proteins** like beef, lamb, chicken, pork, and eggs, along with **vegetables**—steamed, roasted, or sautéed. I also enjoy noodles and other simple meals, but the key for me has been to eat **moderately**. Instead of eating until I'm completely full, I stop when I feel about **70% full**, leaving room for my body to process the food without feeling heavy or sluggish.

This approach has not only helped with **weight management**, but it's also improved my **digestion**. Eating smaller portions allows my body to absorb nutrients more efficiently, and I no longer feel the post-meal lethargy that I used to experience. Drinking water regularly is also an important part of my routine. I've trained myself to drink when my body signals that it's thirsty rather than forcing myself to consume large amounts of water throughout the day.

In addition to water, I enjoy **jasmine green tea** a few times a week, which I find soothing and refreshing. I don't drink coffee regularly, but I'm not opposed to it either. When I do have coffee, I make sure it's **pure**, as coffee has its own set of health benefits, including being rich in **antioxidants**. I've learned to be flexible with my diet, enjoying food without becoming overly restrictive, but always prioritizing how it makes me feel.

4. Simplified Supplementation

In the past, I used to take a wide range of **supplements**—from multivitamins to specific minerals and herbs designed to support thyroid function. But over time, I realized that these supplements were starting to feel heavy on my **liver** and **stomach**, so I've simplified my routine significantly. Now, I focus on just a few key areas, like **iron**, because I have a history of **iron deficiency**.

I typically do an **iron infusion** once every two years, or as needed, based on my **blood test results**. Low iron levels are common with hypothyroidism, and since supplements alone weren't enough to restore my iron levels, infusions have proven to be the most effective way for me to manage this deficiency. This approach allows me to keep my supplement intake minimal while addressing my specific health needs.

5. Natural Sunlight and Grounding: A Holistic Approach to Health

I've also embraced a more **holistic approach** to my overall well-being by focusing on natural sources of healing. Instead of relying on supplements for **vitamin D**, I try to get it through **natural sunlight** whenever possible. There's something incredibly restorative about being outdoors, feeling the warmth of the sun on your skin, and connecting with nature.

I also practice **grounding**—walking barefoot on the earth, whether it's on the grass, the beach, or even in my backyard. There's scientific evidence that grounding can help balance the body's **electrical charge** by connecting with the earth's natural energy. I believe this practice helps me stay **grounded**, both physically and emotionally, and it's a simple, easy way to support my overall health. As we know, **we are energy**, and our bodies function like batteries that need to be recharged through connection with the natural world. I especially like grounding under the Sun light.

6. Gentle Exercise: Walking for Wellness

When it comes to exercise, I've learned that **vigorous workouts** aren't necessary for me to stay healthy. Instead, I prefer **walking**—a simple, yet powerful way to keep my body active without overwhelming it. Walking is an all-in-one exercise that improves

cardiovascular health, boosts **mood**, and enhances **circulation**.

I like to walk **fast**, which gives me the benefits of a cardio workout without the strain of more intense exercise. It's easy to fit into my schedule, whether it's in the early morning, during a break at work, or in the late afternoon. The beauty of walking is that it's accessible to nearly everyone, and you can do it anywhere, anytime. Getting outside for a walk also helps me **stay connected to nature**, which in itself is healing.

7. Sleep: Prioritizing Rest for Recovery

One of the most important parts of my routine is making sure I get enough **sleep**. I aim to go to bed around **10:30 pm**, allowing my body to enter its **deep sleep cycle** during the critical hours between **11 pm and 3 am**, when our internal organs regenerate. Sleep is crucial for anyone managing thyroid disease, as it allows the body to rest, repair, and balance hormone levels.

I've found that having a consistent bedtime helps me wake up feeling more refreshed and energized. Whether it's through calming activities like reading or taking a warm bath, I make sure to unwind in the evening so that I can fall asleep easily and get the restorative rest I need.

8. Consistency and Self-Care: The Pillars of Progress

If there's one thing I've learned through my journey with hypothyroidism, it's that **consistency** is key. Whether it's taking medication, practicing intermittent fasting, or walking daily, the results we achieve are a reflection of the effort we put in. Nothing changes overnight, but small, consistent actions can lead to profound changes in how we feel over time.

I also make it a point to remind myself of the importance of **self-care**. It's easy to get caught up in the demands of life, but making time for ourselves is essential. **Self-discipline** doesn't mean being rigid; it means prioritizing what makes us feel good, both physically and emotionally. As the philosopher **Lao Tzu** once said, *"Conquering others takes force; conquering yourself is true strength."* This quote has become a guiding principle for me—true healing and strength come from within.

Conclusion

Managing hypothyroidism is not just about taking medication; it's about creating a life that supports your health in every possible way. Hypothyroidism affects so many aspects of our well-being, from energy levels and metabolism to mental clarity and mood. While medication is essential, it is only one piece of the puzzle. Through a combination of **balanced nutrition**, **gentle exercise**, **stress management**, and **self-care**, I've been able to find a routine that has transformed the way I feel. This holistic approach has allowed me to feel more in control of my health and, more importantly, it has restored a sense of balance and peace in my daily life.

The journey hasn't always been easy, but it's taught me that healing requires patience, consistency, and a deep commitment to listening to my body. By making small adjustments, staying persistent, and embracing the right lifestyle habits, I've seen significant improvements in my thyroid health and overall well-being. It's not about perfection; it's about progress, and with each step I take, I get closer to feeling like my true self again.

Did you know that our body has an incredible ability to heal and regenerate if we allow it the opportunity to do so? It's something I've come to appreciate more and more through my journey with hypothyroidism. Our bodies are designed to restore balance, but we have to give them the right conditions to make that possible. By focusing on nourishment, movement, and rest, we create an environment that allows healing to happen naturally. This process doesn't happen overnight, but with time and consistency, our bodies can respond in ways we never thought possible.

I encourage you to find what works for you—be patient, be consistent, and most importantly, **listen to your body**. Each of us is unique, and what works for one person may not work for another. That's why it's so important to pay attention to how your body responds to different routines, foods, and practices. Healing is a journey, not a destination. There will be moments when it feels like progress is slow, but don't give up.

Celebrate the small victories along the way—whether it's improved energy, better sleep, or simply feeling more at peace in your daily life. Each positive change is a sign that your body is responding, and those small steps add up over time. The key is to stay committed to yourself and your health. The road to healing from hypothyroidism may be long, but it's worth every effort you put in.

By creating a life that nurtures both your body and your mind, you can thrive with hypothyroidism. It's about more than just managing symptoms—it's about **living fully** and embracing the idea that your health is in your hands. With the right routine, you can live a **full, healthy life**, feeling energized, balanced, and empowered, even while managing hypothyroidism.

Chapter 11: Tips for Thriving with Thyroid Disease – Moving Forward

Living with thyroid disease is a journey that requires ongoing effort, adaptation, and self-awareness. Over time, I've learned that thriving with thyroid disease isn't just about managing symptoms or sticking to medication—it's about creating a lifestyle that supports long-term health and well-being. The goal of this chapter is to share practical steps and insights that have helped me manage my condition, and I hope they will empower you to thrive as well.

1. Practical Steps for Long-Term Management

Successfully managing thyroid disease long-term involves integrating key practices that support both your physical and emotional health. Here are some practical steps that have made a significant difference for me:

- **Consistency with Medication**: One of the most important factors in managing hypothyroidism is staying consistent with medication. Whether you're on **levothyroxine** or **natural desiccated thyroid extract (NDT)**, it's essential to take your medication at the same time each day. This consistency helps regulate hormone levels, and it can prevent the fluctuations that cause symptoms like fatigue or brain fog. Regular blood tests to monitor thyroid hormone levels are also crucial, allowing you and your healthcare provider to adjust your dosage when necessary.

If you are on **NDT**, like I am, I've found that being mindful about the timing of blood tests is important. For example, I feel healthy and balanced on **90 mcg** of NDT, which I believe is the **optimal dose** for me. However, during my last blood test, the results showed that my **T3 levels** were slightly on the high side, and my doctor suggested reducing the dosage. I assured her that I felt well at 90 mcg, and upon reflection, I realized I had taken my thyroid extract just **two hours before** the blood test. This likely skewed the results.

Based on this experience, I recommend doing your **blood tests in the afternoon** if you take your NDT early in the morning. Taking the test too soon after your dose can give you a misleading result, as it may show higher hormone levels that don't accurately reflect how your body is functioning throughout the day. It's important to find a balance with your dosage, based on both **how you feel** and your **blood test results**. Depending on your **height** and **build**, you may require a higher or lower dose than I do, but I would caution against going lower than 90 mcg unless advised by a healthcare provider. As we age, it's also wise to adjust the dose slightly downward, since being **overdosed** with thyroid hormones can lead to other health complications.

- **Diet and Nutrition**: What you eat has a profound effect on your thyroid health. Following an **anti-inflammatory diet**, rich in whole foods like vegetables, lean proteins, and healthy fats, helps support the thyroid and reduce inflammation in the body. I've found that eliminating processed foods and focusing on nutrient-dense meals has improved my energy levels and overall well-being. If possible, try to include iodine-rich foods, such as seaweed and eggs, and ensure you're getting enough selenium through foods like Brazil nuts.

- **Supplements**: While I used to rely on various supplements to support my thyroid health, I've simplified my routine over time. In fact, I haven't taken any of these supplements for about a year now and feel fine. However, some patients find key supplements beneficial, particularly **selenium**, which is crucial for the conversion of T4 to T3. **Vitamin D** is another important nutrient, especially if you're not getting enough sunlight. **Omega-3 fatty acids** can help reduce inflammation, which is particularly useful in autoimmune thyroid conditions like Hashimoto's. Even though I no longer take these supplements myself, it's always a good idea to consult with your healthcare provider before adding or changing any supplements in your regimen.

- **Hydration and Detoxification**: Staying hydrated is often overlooked, but it's vital for maintaining good thyroid function. Drinking enough water helps flush toxins from the body and supports digestion, which is often slower in hypothyroidism. Additionally, supporting your liver—your body's main detox organ—is important for thyroid health. I recommend incorporating liver-supportive foods like garlic, turmeric, and leafy greens to help with natural detoxification.

- **Exercise and Movement**: Regular movement is key for boosting metabolism and improving energy levels, particularly for those managing hypothyroidism. It doesn't have to be intense—gentle exercises like walking, yoga, or swimming can do wonders for maintaining muscle mass and stimulating blood flow. For me, walking has become an essential part of my routine. Not only does it improve my physical health, but it also provides an opportunity to de-stress and reflect.

- **Stress Management**: Managing stress is crucial for thyroid health. Chronic stress can worsen symptoms, and for many thyroid patients, stress is a trigger for flare-ups. That's why it's important to make stress management a priority. Whether it's through **meditation, deep breathing exercises**, or simply taking time out of your day to relax, finding ways to reduce stress will help balance your hormones and improve your quality of life.

2. Balancing Medication, Lifestyle, and Mental Health

While medication is a vital part of managing thyroid disease, it's only one aspect of the larger picture. To truly thrive, it's important to find balance between your medication, lifestyle habits, and mental health.

- **Personalizing Your Approach**: Each person's experience with thyroid disease is different, which means there's no one-size-fits-all solution. What worked for me might not work for you, so it's essential to develop a routine that's tailored to your unique needs. Whether it's adjusting your diet, finding the right exercise routine, or experimenting with different supplements, be open to trying new things and seeing what makes you feel your best.

- **Listening to Your Body**: One of the most valuable lessons I've learned is the importance of listening to my body. There will be days when you feel great, and there will be days when your energy is low or your symptoms flare up. Learning to tune into your body's signals and adjusting accordingly is crucial for long-term success. Don't be afraid to rest when you need it, and don't push yourself too hard when your body is telling you to slow down.

- **Self-Care for Mental Health**: Mental health is often overlooked when managing thyroid disease, but it's just as important as physical health. Hypothyroidism, in particular, can lead to feelings of depression, anxiety, and brain fog. That's why it's essential to incorporate mental health practices into your routine. Whether it's seeing a therapist, practicing mindfulness, or simply taking time each day to unwind, prioritizing your mental well-being will help you stay balanced.

- **Regular Check-ins with Healthcare Providers**: It's important to have regular check-ins with your healthcare provider to monitor your thyroid levels and adjust your treatment plan as needed. As thyroid hormone levels can change over time, having a supportive and knowledgeable healthcare provider is key to ensuring that your medication and supplements are properly balanced. Always communicate openly about how you're feeling—both physically and emotionally—so that adjustments can be made.

- **Adapting as Needed**: Thyroid disease is not static, and neither is your routine. There may be times when your body changes, and you need to adapt your approach. Don't be afraid to make changes to your routine if something stops working or if you feel you need to try something new. Flexibility is important, and it's okay to adjust as your body and health evolve over time.

3. Words of Encouragement

Living with thyroid disease can feel overwhelming at times, but I want to reassure you that it is possible to thrive. Managing this condition requires patience, resilience, and a commitment to taking care of yourself, but the journey is worth it.

- **Embracing the Journey**: Your thyroid health journey is unique to you, and it's important to embrace it. There will be ups and downs, but each step forward is progress. Take pride in the small victories—whether it's improved energy, a better mood, or even just a good day where your symptoms are less intense.

- **Staying Resilient**: Resilience is key. There will be setbacks, and that's okay. Healing isn't linear, but with persistence and self-compassion, you can navigate through the tough times. Remember that you are stronger than you realize, and each challenge you face is an opportunity to learn more about your body and how to care for it.

- **Community and Support**: Don't underestimate the power of support. Whether it's through family, friends, or online communities of people going through the same struggles, having a support system can make all the difference. You don't have to face this journey alone, and sharing your experiences with others can provide comfort and encouragement.

- **Finding Your Strength**: Living with thyroid disease takes strength, and you should celebrate that strength every day. You've navigated complex challenges, and you continue to show up for yourself despite the difficulties. That in itself is an achievement. Every step you take toward better health, no matter how small, is something to be proud of.

Conclusion

Managing thyroid disease is a lifelong journey, but it's one that can lead to incredible growth, resilience, and self-awareness. By balancing medication, lifestyle, and mental health, you can take control of your health and thrive. Remember that healing is a process, and it's important to be patient with yourself along the way.

Take the time to develop a routine that works for you, stay connected with your healthcare providers, and don't be afraid to advocate for your needs. With the right approach, you can live a full, healthy life while managing thyroid disease—and most importantly, you can continue moving forward with hope, strength, and confidence.

Chapter 12: Conclusion – Reflecting on the Journey

As I reach the conclusion of this book, I find myself reflecting on the journey I've travelled, not just in managing my thyroid disease, but in rediscovering what it means to truly care for my body, mind, and spirit. Living with both hyperthyroidism and hypothyroidism has brought a range of challenges, some of which seemed insurmountable at times. But looking back now, I can see how each step along the way has led me to a place of greater strength, resilience, and understanding.

When I was first diagnosed, I never could have imagined how much this journey would teach me. The initial confusion, frustration, and physical discomfort felt overwhelming. I struggled with the symptoms, the medication adjustments, and the emotional toll that thyroid disease can bring. There were moments when I questioned if I'd ever regain a sense of normalcy, or if I would always feel stuck between managing one health issue after another.

But through the years, I've learned that healing doesn't follow a straight line. There are ups and downs, setbacks and breakthroughs. I've come to understand that managing thyroid disease is not about finding a quick fix, but about learning to navigate my health in a way that's sustainable and supportive for the long haul. Each small victory along the way, whether it was finally finding the right medication, making dietary changes that boosted my energy, or simply learning to manage stress better, has been part of my larger journey toward healing.

Empowerment and Proactivity: Taking Charge of Your Health

One of the most valuable lessons I've learned is that we are our own best advocates. While doctors and specialists play an important role in diagnosing and treating thyroid disease, it's up to us to take an active role in our own health. Throughout my journey, I've had to make difficult decisions—whether it was opting for surgery, seeking alternative treatments, or challenging the standard protocols I was being offered.

I've learned the importance of staying informed, asking questions, and never being afraid to seek second opinions. The medical system doesn't always have the answers, and it's up to us to explore different paths to find what truly works. Whether it was researching natural desiccated thyroid extract, finding alternative doctors, or learning about lifestyle changes that could support my thyroid health, I realized that my health is ultimately in my hands.

Being proactive is key. This means staying on top of regular check-ups, advocating for the right treatments, and being mindful of the signals your body is sending. Throughout this journey, I've had to adjust my approach multiple times—whether it was tweaking my medication dosage, changing my diet, or incorporating new stress management techniques. The point is, managing thyroid disease is an ongoing process that requires flexibility, patience, and a willingness to advocate for yourself.

There is power in **taking charge of your health**. It's about realizing that you are in control, even when it feels like your body is working against you. By making informed decisions, listening to your body, and staying persistent, you can create a path that supports your long-term well-being.

Finding Hope: Healing and Balance are Possible

If there's one message I want to leave you with, it's this: healing is possible. No matter how difficult your journey has been, no matter how long you've struggled with the symptoms and challenges of thyroid disease, there is always hope. It's easy to feel discouraged when progress feels slow, but I've learned that every step forward, no matter how small, brings you closer to a place of balance.

For me, healing didn't happen overnight. It took years of trial and error, research, and persistence. There were times when I felt like I was going backward, especially when dealing with the transition from hyperthyroidism to hypothyroidism after my thyroidectomy. I had to relearn what my body needed, find the right balance between medication, diet, and lifestyle, and, most importantly, I had to learn to be patient with myself.

Healing requires **consistency** and **patience**. You may not see immediate results, but that doesn't mean progress isn't happening. Over time, I've come to appreciate the small victories—the days when I have more energy, the moments when my mental clarity improves, or when I manage to handle stress with more ease. These are all signs that healing is unfolding, even when it feels slow.

One of the most empowering realizations I had during this journey is that **our bodies are designed to heal**. Did you know that if we give our bodies the right conditions—through proper nutrition, rest, stress management, and balanced medication—our bodies can regenerate and heal themselves? It's something I've come to deeply believe. Our bodies are powerful, and with the right approach, we can create the space for healing to happen naturally.

It's important to stay **hopeful**, even when things feel difficult. Finding the right balance between thyroid management and overall wellness takes time, but I want to assure you that balance is achievable. You may need to make adjustments along the way, but with persistence, you can regain control of your health and start feeling more like yourself again.

Words of Encouragement

Living with thyroid disease is undoubtedly challenging, and if you're reading this, you've already demonstrated incredible strength by seeking out knowledge and taking control of your health. There will be days when you feel frustrated or overwhelmed, and that's completely normal. But remember, healing is not a race—it's a journey. Each step you take, no matter how small, brings you closer to finding the balance and wellness you deserve.

I encourage you to remain steadfast in advocating for yourself. Your health is your greatest asset, and you have every right to question, challenge, and push for the care that best suits your needs. Trust your instincts—no one knows your body better than you do. If something doesn't feel right, don't hesitate to explore new options or seek second opinions. The more informed and empowered you are, the better equipped you'll be to navigate the complexities of thyroid disease.

Be patient with yourself along the way. Healing isn't always linear, and it's okay to take things one day at a time. Celebrate the victories, no matter how small—whether it's feeling a little more energized, sleeping better, or finding moments of peace in your day. These are signs that you're making progress, and they're worth acknowledging.

You are not alone. There's a community of individuals who understand exactly what you're going through, and they stand with you in solidarity. Sharing your story, connecting with others, and offering support can make a world of difference. We all walk this path together, and together, we find strength.

In the end, thriving with thyroid disease isn't just possible—it's within your reach. It's about finding the right balance in your routines, supporting your body through thoughtful care, and believing in your ability to heal. I hope that this book has given you not only practical tools but also a sense of hope and reassurance.

Healing takes time, but you are capable, and a vibrant, healthy life is waiting for you on the other side.

Conclusion

Managing thyroid disease is a lifelong journey, but it's also a journey filled with growth, strength, and self-discovery. By taking control of your health, staying proactive, and finding balance, you can overcome the challenges of thyroid disease and live a fulfilling, empowered life. Healing is possible, and every small step brings you closer to the health and well-being you deserve.

Final Words to My Readers

As I close the final page of this book, I want to take a moment to acknowledge you, the reader. If you've made it this far, you've likely faced your own challenges with thyroid disease, whether you're newly diagnosed, have been living with the condition for years, or are supporting a loved one through their journey. I hope that in sharing my story, you've found encouragement, insights, and perhaps even a sense of connection.

Writing this book has been both cathartic and deeply personal. I've poured into these pages the lessons I've learned through trial and error, the moments of doubt and fear, as well as the breakthroughs that have brought me closer to balance and healing. I didn't know when I first started this journey just how much it would teach me—not just about thyroid disease, but about resilience, self-advocacy, and the power of hope.

I want to leave you with this thought: **You are stronger than you realize**. Living with a chronic condition like thyroid disease can be overwhelming, but you have the strength within you to overcome its challenges. Every step you take toward better health, no matter how small, is a victory. Celebrate those moments. Healing is not linear, and it may feel slow at times, but trust in your body's ability to heal and in your own ability to persevere.

Take everything you've learned—whether from this book, your doctors, or your own experience—and create a path that works for you. Be patient with yourself, stay informed, and never be afraid to advocate for your needs. Your health journey is uniquely yours, and it's important to find what makes you feel your best.

Remember, you are not alone. There are others walking this same path, and together, we can navigate the complexities of thyroid disease with greater understanding and compassion.

Thank you for allowing me to share my journey with you. My hope is that it has provided you with some comfort, guidance, and a renewed sense of hope for your own health. Stay strong, stay empowered, and most importantly, **stay hopeful**—because healing and balance are always within reach.

With gratitude,
Brin De Bellis